Hygiene and Sanitation.

Hygiene and Sanitation

("Gesundheitsbüchlein")

A popular Manual to Hygiene.

Compiled

by

The Imperial Board of Health.
(Kaiserliches Gesundheitsamt.)

With figures in the Text and two coloured engravings.

Ninth, revised edition.

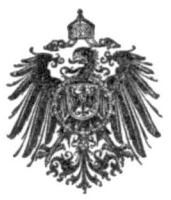

BERLIN
Julius Springer
1904.

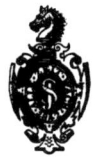

ISBN 978-3-642-48517-6   ISBN 978-3-642-48584-8 (eBook)
DOI 10.1007/978-3-642-48584-8

Softcover reprint of the hardcover 1st edition 1904

Preface.

The spreading of a more general culture, which forms the basis of professional perfection has the effect, that certain provinces of knowledge, which in former times were reserved to the professional man only are becoming the property of every educated man. This „broadening" of knowledge does not at all mean a restriction of science for the professional „Savants". On the contrary. They are enabled to follow the progress of science more closely by receiving a more careful training for their profession, and they can obtain better results with the help of a more educated public, when called upon to make a practical use of their professional knowledge or skill.

This development took place in a very marked degree with regard to the science of Hygiene, public Hygiene as well as private sanitation.

An epidemic disease, cholera for instance, can be fought more successfully when the public intelligently assist the authorites, than when it obstructs the work of the doctors, or when it threatens or even ill-treats them; as happened in some parts of Europe a few years ago. A private person can be restored to health much quicker, if the patient and those, who are near him follow intelligently the orders of the medical adviser and assist him with their knowledge of Hygiene, than if they do not understand the orders, or if they treat them with indifference.

One ought to be able to say, or to suppose at least at the present time, that every educated person has some knowledge of the science of Hygiene and of sanitation; we might also expect, that the tuition and instruction in the higher schools will gradually extend in that direction. If a future generation goes even further, so much the better.

The Imperial Board of Health (Gesundheitsamt) always considered as its first aim the promotion and furtherance, the practical realization of scientific doctrines. It considers itself therefore particularly called upon to select from the whole realm of the science of Hygiene those matters, which ought to be known everywhere and to state them in a manner intelligible to all.

These are the considerations, to which this little „Gesundheitsbüchlein" owes its origin. The director as well as the members of the Board of Health cooperated at it.

They also received valuable help from others, for which the Department tenders its thanks. May this little book be received in the same spirit, in which its authors wrote it; as a contribution towards the furtherance of the well-being of the people, which at present forms the guiding principle for our statesmen. Its importance has been recognized by H. M. the Emperor, and we Germans look with just pride upon the beneficial resolutions as the consequence of such high-minded assistance.

Berlin, July 1894.

Contents.

	Page
Introduction. The value of Hygiene	1—3

A. The structure of the human body; the action and the uses of its organs

The constituent parts of the human body.

1. Description of the parts of the body. 2. Bones and cartilage. 3. Ligaments, Joints. 4. Muscles, sinews. 5. Glands. 6. The skin; the mucous membranes . . . . 4—6

Some parts of the body and their functions.

7. General division of the body. 8. The Head, the Face, the facial cavities. 9. The Trunk; the cavities of the Trunk. 10. The Upper Limbs. 11. The Lower Limbs. 12. The viscera of the thorax. 13. The Lungs and Breathing. 14. The Larynx; the voice and speech. 15. The Blood; the bloodvessels; the heart and the circulation of the Blood. 16. Relations of the circulation of the blood to respiration. 17. Lymph, Lymph-vessels and Lymph-glands. 18. Viscera of the Abdomen. 19. The stomach, the oesophagus, the intestinal canal, the mesenteric and the Netz. 20. The liver, gall and Pancreas. 21. Digestion (Stoffwechsel). 22. The head of the Body. Fever. 23. Urine; the Kidneys and the Urinary canals. 24. The Spleen. 25. The action of the nerves. The Brain, and the spinal marrow. 26. The organs of sense. 27. The sense of sight. The eyes. 28. The sense of Hearing. The Ears. 29. Taste; Smell; Touch. 30. Sleep. 31. Propagation . . . . 6—34

B. The necessaries of life for the individual man.

32. The necessaries of man's life in general 35

I. The Air.

33. The atmosphere and its composition. 34. Nitrogen, oxygen and carbonic acid of the air. 35. Moisture and Heat of the

VIII   Contents.

                                                                   Page
air. 36. Movement of the air-deposits. 37. The pressure of
the air. 38. Contamination of air. 39. The climate . . . . 35—42

II. Water.

40. Importance of water. 41. Drinking water; its necessary properties. 42. The source of water. Rainwater. Cisterns. 43. Subterranean water and springs. 44. Spring-water pipes. Well-Machinery. 45. Surface Water. 46. Artificial purification of the surface water. Filters. 47. Sea-water. 48. Mineral water. 49. Use of water in removing dirt. 50. Auxiliaries of water for cleansing. Cleansing of the body and the care of skin and hair. 51. Baths and water cures . . . . 42—54

III. Food.

52. Necessity of food. 53. Composition of food. 54. Food and nutritive substances. 55. Choice of food. 56. Calculation of daily diet. 57. Preparation of food. Spices and other provisions. 58. Manner of taking food. Care of the mouth and the Teeth . . . . 54—61

The Means of Nourishment.

59. Selection of food as a calculation of our diet. 60. Corn and flour. 61. Preparation of flour. Pastry. 62. Different kinds of bread. 63. Cakes and tarts. 64. The different kinds of Grain. 65. Pulses. 66. Oil products. 67. Potatoes. Fresh vegetables. 68. The fresh or green vegetables. 69. Fungi and Mushrooms. 70. Fruit. 71. Sugar. 72. Honey. 73. Confectionary. 74. Food from the animal kingdom. 75. Milk. 76. Formation of cream and souring of milk. 77. Preserved milk. 78. Adulterations of milk. 79. Butter. 80. Cheese. 81. Eggs. 82. Meat. 83. Flesh of diseased animals. Parasites of meat. 84. Decayed meat. Inspection of meat. 85. Preparation of meat. Boiled meat. Meat soup. Stewing; Baking and Roasting. 86. Preserved meat. 87. Food, manufactured from meat. 88. Fishes. 89. Crustaceae and shell-fish. 90. Seasonings. Salt; vegetable acids; vinegar. 91. Spices. 92. Refreshments. 93. Alcohol. 94. Wine. 95. Beer. 96. Brandy. Liqueurs. 97. Coffee; tea; cocoa. 98. Tobacco. 99. Food utensils and food dishes. 100. Storage of food . . . . 61—102

IV. Clothing.

101. Clothing as a protection against cooling. 102. Clothing as a protection against dampness. 103. Selection of the material for clothing. 104. Colour; shape and fastenings of garments. 105. Clothing for the neck. 106. Constriction of the body by

the clothing, or by the way of fastening it. 107. Garters; Boots and shoes. 108. Covering of the head. 109. The Bed. 110. Cleanliness of clothing and bedding . . . . 102—109

V. The dwelling.

111. Purpose of the dwelling. 112. Subsoil and site of the house. 113. Building-materials. 114. Drainage and drying of the House. The roof. 115. The final touches on a house. Floors. Walls. 116. Utilization of dwelling-rooms. Air-space. Plan of the dwelling. 117. Ventilation. 118. Purpose of heating. Requisites of a heating apparatus. 119. Fireplaces and iron stoves. 120. Filled stoves; stoves with hoods. 121. Earthenware stoves. 122. Collective heating by air, water or steam. 123. Protection of the house from heat. 124. Brightness. Natural lighting. 125. Artificial lighting. Candles. Oil- and Petroleum lamps. 126. Gas lighting. Electric light. 127. Protection of the eyes by shades. 128. Cleanliness in the dwelling. Removal of refuse. 129. Removal of human excreta. 130. Height of the dwelling. Attics and cellar dwellings (basements). 131. Articles for use in the dwellings . . 109—128

VI. Exercise and Recreation.

132. Exercise and Recreation . . . . 128—129

C. Man in his relation to society.

133. Communities. Public Hygiene 130

I. Settlements.

134. Importance of settlements for health. 135. The Locality 136. The removal of refuse in settlements. 137. The final destruction of refuse. 138. Removal of waste water from factories. 139. Street cleaning. 140. The supply of water. 141. The "modus" of laying out a settlement. 142. Dispersion of smoke, and other atmospheric impurities. The avoiding of nuisances from factories. 143. Civilization and prosperity of the people. 144. Provisions for the sale of food. Supervision of crowds, theatres, assembly rooms, pleasure resorts etc. 145. Provision for the poor and sick. 146. Funerals. 147. Inspection of corpses. Disposal of corpses of persons, who have died of infectious diseases. 148. Removal of dead animals . 131—144

II. Commerce.

149. Objects of commerce. Means of communication. 150. Travelling. 151. Prevention of the spread of infectious diseases by traffic. 152. Closure of frontiers; Quarantines. 153. Mea-

Contents.

sures against the spreading of epidemics in Germany. 154. Other risks through goods traffic .... 144—148

III. Education.

155. General influence of education. 156. Mortality of infants. 157. The foods for infants. 158. Baths. Children's clothing. Necessity of fresh air. Eye-diseases of newly-born infants. Sleep. Causes of children's crying. 159. Cutting the teeth. Development of speech. Standing and walking. 160. Awakening of intellect; Kindergarten. 161. School hours; duties of the government, the masters, physician-teachers and parents. 162. The schoolhouse and the schoolroom. 163. Relation between the lighting of the schoolroom and the origin of short-sight. 164. Schoolforms; curvatures of the spine. 165. The alleged over pressure of pupils. Injudicious division of school-lessons. 166. Mode of life during the period of life, when the child is compelled to school-attendance. 167. Development and protection of the body in the schools. Gymnastic training. 168. Capacity of pupils. 169. Girl's education in particular .... 149—160

IV. Employment and Wages.

170. Advantages and disadvantages of special occupations in relation to health. Factory inspectors. 171. Importance of choice of profession — Prevention of weakly persons from entering in labourious occupations. Limitation of hours of labour for women and children. 172. Duration of daily work. 173. Injuries to health by overworking certain parts of the body. 174. Influence of the weather. Effect of very great heat. 175. Dust disease. 176. Noxious gases. 177. Poisoning by metals or Phosphorus. 178. Accidents. 179. Precautionary measures against accidents during work. 180. Statistics of illnesses and deaths in different trades and occupations . . 161—169

D. Dangers to health from external influences.

I. Injuries to health from weather and climate.

181. The cause and various classes of colds. 182. Precautions against "colds". 183. Frost-bites. 184. Treatment of frost bitten persons. 185. Heat-stroke; sun-stroke; lightning stroke. 186. Climate and seasons .... 170—175

II. Infectious diseases.

a) In general.

187. Nature and manner of spreading infectious diseases. 188. Disease germs. 189. Preliminary conditions of infection. 190. Pre-

Contents. XI

ventive measures against infectious diseases. 191. Combating infectious diseases. 192. Course of illnesses, arising from infection. 193. Fever .... 175—184

b) Some infectious diseases.

194. Acute eruptive diseases. 195. Measles and German measles. 196. Scarlet fever (Scarlatina). 197. Small-pox. 198. Vaccination. 199. Chicken-pox. 200. Typhus. Spotted fever. 201. Remittent fever. 202. Typhoid fever. 203. Gastric fever. Catarrh of the stomach and intestines. Diarrhoea. 204. Cholera. 205. Dysentery. 206. Diphtheria, Croup, Tonsillitis. 207. Whooping-cough. 208. Influenza. 209. Inflammation of the lungs. Pleurisy. Peritonitis. 210. Epidemic stiff-neck. Inflammation of the cerebral membrane. 211. Intermittent fever. 212. The Plague. 213. Yellow fever. 214. Wound diseases. 215. Inflammation; Suppuration; Whitlow; furuncle, Carbuncle. 216. Inflammation of the lymph vessels. Inflammation of the lymph glands. Purulent and putrid fever. Puerperal fever. 217. Erysipelas and gangrene. 218. Tetanus. 219. Contagious diseases of the eye. 220. Contagious animal diseases. 221. Hydrophobia. 222. Anthrax. Glanders. 223. Other diseases of animals, which may be communicated to man. 224. Syphilis. 225. Leprosy. 226. Tuberculosis. 227. Individual forms of tuberculosis. 228. Scrofula. Curable nature of tuberculosis. 229. Dissemination of tuberculosis and preventive measures against it .... 185—213

III. Other diseases.

220. Diseases of the nerves and the brain. Disorders in the formation of blood, and the development of the body. 231. Tumours and Cancer .... 213—216

IV. Accidents.

232. Frequency of accidents. Value of the first assistance offered. Various kinds of accidents. 233. Wounds and bleedings. 234. Fractures of bones. Dislocations and sprains. 235. Burns and corrosions. 236. Poisoning and intoxication. 237. Fainting fits and cramps. 238. Coma. 239. Artificial respiration. Conduct in saving from suffocation. Foreign substances in the natural apertures of the body .... 217—231

Supplement.

Preliminary knowledge for nursing the sick.

240. Importance of nursing. 231. The sick-room. 242. The sick-bed. 243. Care of the patient's Body. Bedsores.

244. Watching by the sick. Conduct of the nurse. 245. Sleep and breathing of the patient. 246. Bleeding. 247. Heartbeat; Pulse; Temperature of the body. 248. Natural excretions of the patient. Injections and enemas. 249. Vomiting. Attention to bandages. Nourishment of the invalid. 250. Giving of medicine. 251. Painting. Massage. Embrocation. 252. Mustard-plasters and blisters. 253. Ice-bags. Cold bandages. 254. Cold douches and swathings. Moistwarm bandages. Dry heat. 255. Baths. Sweating cures. 256. Transport of the sick . . . . 232—243

Introduction.

The value of Hygiene. (Gesundheitspflege.)

Man's health is a precious good. Its loss causes injury and harm not only to the individual person, but also to the community.

The individual, whose health is impaired feels discomfort or pain; he loses the power for working, the ability for earning money and of enjoying life. He is compelled to spend large sums of money for the recovery of his health; sorrows, distress and misery for himself and his family may be the results of bad health.

The Community loses through the diminution of the working power of the individual citizen and incurs besides expenditure for the support of the sick. In cases of contagious diseases sick persons are moreover a cause of danger to their neighbours.

We can make an estimate of the economic losses, which are caused by illnesses from the statistical returns of the working men's sick clubs in Germany. In the year 1898 there were more than three million cases of sickness out of a total membership of $8\frac{3}{4}$ million members of the clubs, each case lasting on the average about 17.7 days. The clubs spent on medical expenses for their members about 128 millions mark. As we may safely assume, that among the other 45 million inhabitants of Germany (of whom 25 millions belong to the age, in which they can earn money) cases of illness were not less numerous and not of shorter duration, than among the members of the clubs, the estimate of expenses spent caused by sickness in the German Empire during the year 1898 cannot be put down at less than 600 millions of mark. This sum does not include the loss through stoppage or cessation of work.

The scope of the science of Hygiene is the preservaticn and promotion of human health; its task consists therefore first of all in the prevention, restriction and removal of sicknesses and diseases; in the conservation and prolongation of the power of earning money, and of the prolongation of man's life itself.

To the observance of the rules of the science of Hygiene we owe the fact, that the number of cases of sickness in the German army, which amounted in 1868 to 1496 and between 1879 and 1882 to 1147.5 per 1000 soldiers decreased during the five years 1892—1897 to 790 per 1000 men. When we consider, that in round numbers the German army consists of half a million soldiers, we find that during the years 1892 to 1897 the number of cases of illness decreased in each year by 178750 compared with the number of cases of sickness in each year during the period of 1879—1882.

The decline in the death-rate in the general civil community can easily be proved as soon as the rules of the sanitary science are better obeyed, and the economic gain caused by such higher sanitary supervision can easily be shown by the following example. According to von Pettenkofer's investigations the proportion of cases of death to cases of illness in Munich before the year 1877 was 1 : 34; each case of illness averaging about 20 days. If the mortality in Munich since 1877 dereased in such a proportion, that of 1000 inhabitants duriug the period between 1895 and 1900 on the average about *9 persons less* died in each year than before 1877, then there were in Munich with its 425 000 (in round numbers) inhabitants during the period of 1895—1900 in every year 3825 less cases of death than would have occurred before 1877 according to the mortality then prevailing. The inhabitants of Munich have therefore been spared during the years 1895—1900 in every year $3825 \times 34 \times 20 =$ i. e. $2\frac{1}{2}$ million days of sickness, compared to the days of sickness before 1877. Assuming that the expenses of each day of sickness for nursing, medicine etc. come to $1\frac{3}{4}$ mark, we find that the city of Munich has been saved an expenditure of $3\frac{3}{4}$ millions of mark in every year through the decrease of the number of days of illness; thus making a saving of 8 to 9 mark per head of its population, or 44 mark for each family of five persons.

The *suitable care*, *nursing* and *treatment* of the patients is also one of the aims of the science of Hygiene, besides the prevention of sicknesses. A quick restoration of health may be attained in the shortest time and in the surest way by proper treatment. In this connection the clubs and other similar institutions are of great importance. They alleviate the lot of the patient and of his family; they contribute to diminish the number of days of illness and thus restrict in the most efficacious manner the lenght of time, during which the work of the patient and his earnings are interrupted:

Some knowledge of the nature and of the functions of the human body is necessary for the purpose of enabling us to appreciate fully the value and the demands of Hygiene. The human body forms after all the principal aim of the science of Hygiene.

A. The structure of the human body; the action and the uses of its organs.

The constituent parts of the human body.

§ 1. Description of the parts of the body. We have to distinguish between the *hard portions* of the body, its *soft* and the liquid constituents parts. The hard are the *bones*, the *cartilage* and the teeth. The bones are united by strong ligaments; the totality of the bones of the human body is called *the skeleton.*

To the soft parts of the body belong the *skin*, the *adipose tissues*, the *muscles*, the *entrails* (viscera) the *bloodvessels* and the *nerves*. The boodvessels and the nerves are spread through all parts of the human body; the fatty tissue is found principally immediately under the skin, but it also passes through the muscles and the viscera.

Among the liquid constituents the *blood* has the greatest importance.

§ 2. Bones and cartilage. The bones, of which we know over 200 in the human body are partly hollow tubes, which contain in their interior a soft mass, rich in blood, called the *bone marrow*. Besides these reed-bones there are also flat bones, for instance the external bones of the skull and spongy bones, like the vertebræ. Every bone is surrounded by a thin fine membrane, called the *Periosteum*.

Many bones change at their ends into cartilage, which is an elastic mass, similar to the substance of the bone, but less hard. Independent cartilages unconnected with a bone are to be found in the *larynx* and in the auricle.

§ 3. Ligaments, Joints. Bones are ordinarily connected together by strong ligaments; such a connection is called *a joint*, if it permits a movement of one bone towards the other.

Each joint represents a hermetically (air tight) closed capsule, formed of masses of ligaments, in which rest the ends of several bones, covered by a flat cartilaginous mass; it contains a small portion of a mucous thread-like fluid, the *joint grease* (synovia) which facilitates the gliding of the ends of the bones over one another. While some joints, for instance the middle finger-joint permit movement in one plane only, other joints for instance the shoulder joint (the capular) permit much more extended movements in various directions.

§ 4. **Muscles, sinews.** The muscles bring about the movements in the body and in its component parts. They constitute the principal mass of the flesh, they are composed of bundles of fibre and possess the property of shortening themselves by contraction and of reverting again to their longer form from the contracted state by relaxation.

The muscles ordinarily lie between the skin and the bones, and are joined to the latter by means of ribbon-like bands, the sinews. By its contraction the muscle, like a stretched band of india rubber gets shorter and thereby causes those parts of the body to come nearer to one another, to which its ends are fastened. If (for example) in the outstretched arm the fore-muscle of the upper arm contracts, the lower arm thereby is brought nearer to the upper arm; that means, that a bending of the arm at the elbow-joint follows. If the same muscle then relaxes, it gets lengthened again and the arm returns from the bent into the outstretched position, as soon as the hind muscle of the upper arm contracts.

§ 5. **Glands.** Some of the organs, which belong to the soft parts of the body secrete fluids from their tissues or from the blood which flows through them; these fluids are either used during the different functions of the body, as for instance the gastric juice in the process of digestion, or they leave the body and remove matter which can no longer be used in the body, as the urine, secreted in the kidneys. These organs are called *glands*. They generally possess one or more excretory ducts, through which is discharged the secreted fluid. Besides the large glands, to which for instance the liver belongs, there are minutely small glands, which are hardly visible without the aid of a magnifying-glass, like the perspiratory glands. The secretion from the glands may be a thin fluid like the urine, or slimy like the saliva or viscous like the ear-wax.

Some other organs, which secrete nothing externally, are also called glands; for instance the lymphatic glands (cf. § 17).

§ 6. The skin; the mucous membranes. Our *skin* forms the outer (external) covering of our body; it consists of two layers, the more tender *epidermis* and the corium under it. The *epidermis* is covered with fine hair, which in some parts of the body, as for instance on the head attain considerable length and thickness. The back of the ends of the fingers and of the toes is specially protected by horny, non sensitive substances, called *nails*. In the derma (corium, harder skin) we find the skin-glands, small tube-like structures, the aperture of which, opening on the surface are called the *pores* of the skin. Some skin-glands secrete a fatty mass, the skin grease, which gives to the skin its flexibility and lustre; by other skin-glands is secreted the *sweat*, the well-known watery and salty fluid.

The skin changes at the natural openings of the body into a similar covering, which is called the mucous membrane. This transition can be plainly seen at the lips and also at the eyelids, where the boundary line between the skin and the mucous membrane is specially marked by the eyelashes.

The *mucous membrane* covers the cavities which are connected with the natural apertures of the body (nostrils, larynx, mouth, œsophagus, stomach, intestines); it is of a more tender construction than the external skin, has a reddish appearance as it allows the bloodvessels to be seen through, which are filled with red blood. The surface of the mucous membranes is moist and slippery, owing to a mucus which is secreted by microscopically small glands.

Some parts of the Body and their Functions.

§ 7. General division of the body. The human body is divided into the *head*, the *trunk* and the *limbs*. (Fig. 1.)

In the head we distinguish between the *skull* and the *face*. The skull, approaching in shape that of a hemisphere encloses the *cranial cavity*, in which is situated the *brain*. In the skull we distinguish in front the *forehead*, on the top the *crown of the head*, on both sides the *temples* and at the back the *occiput*.

The crown, the occiput and parts of the temples are

Some parts of the Body and their Functions. 7

covered with *hair*. In the face we notice the *eyes*, the *nose*, the *mouth*, the *cheeks* and the *chin*. On the boundary line between the skull and the face are the *ears*.

The *Trunk* is divided into the *neck*, the backpart of which is called the *nape;* the *breast*, the *belly*, the *back*, the *loins*, and the *pelvis*, the sides of which are the *hips*. The furrow which separates the trunk in front from the upper thigh is called *bend of the groin*. The trunk contains two large cavities, which are filled with *entrails*, the *thorax* and the *abdomen*. Among the limbs we distinguish the upper limbs or *arms* from the lower limbs or *legs*.

§ 8. The Head, the Face, the facial cavities. (Fig. 2.) The head is composed of the bones of the skull and of the facial bones, which are covered with soft tissues; these bones are nearly all joined together immovably firm. The *lower jaw* alone, which belongs to the facial bones possesses moveableness; the ends of its joints are situated in front of the ears; their movements, in chewing for instance can be felt by placing the finger on that spot. Other facial bones are the two bones of the nose, which join to form the osseous bridge of the nose, the Zygoma or *cheekbones* and the two *bones of the upper jaw*.

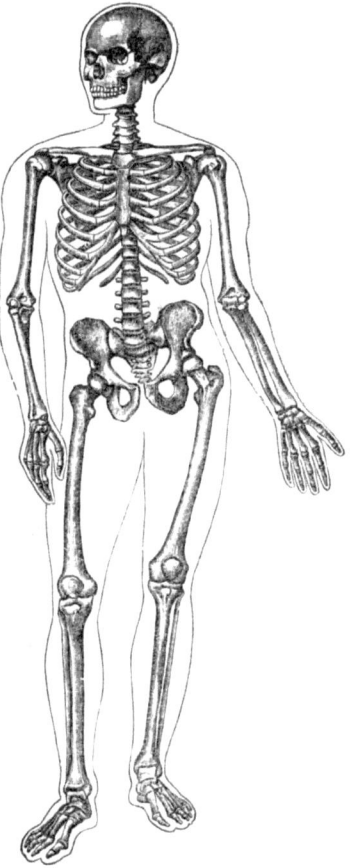

Fig. 1. Skeleton.

The facial bones form partly by themselves partly with the skull as well as with the cartilages and tissues the two orbits (cavities of the eyes) the *cavity* of the *nose* and the *oral cavity*.

8   A. The structure of the human body.

The cavities of the eyes, which are formed only by bones are widely opened in front, extend back deeply into the head and become narrower, as they recede inwards and backwards. From their hindmost part a small, round opening, through which

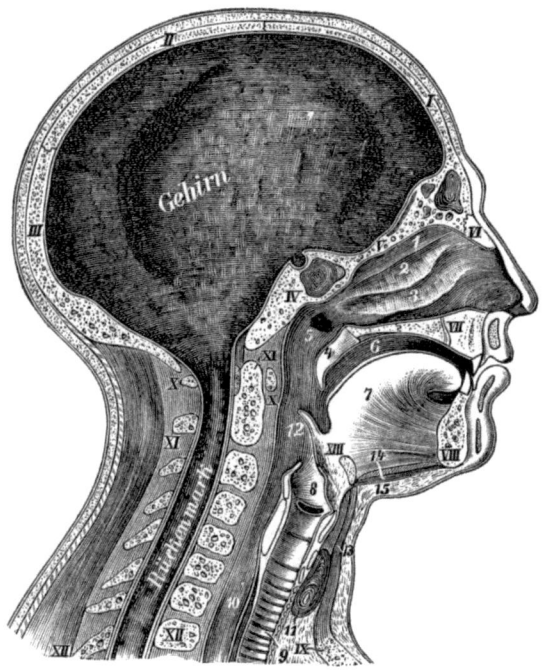

Fig. 2. *Head and Neck.*

I—V. Bones of the skull. (*I* Frontal Bone. *II* Parietal Bone, *III* Occipital Bone. *IV* Sphenoid Bone. *V* Optic Bone.) *VI* Nasal Bone. *VII* Upper Jaw. *VIII* Lower Jaw. *IX* Breastbone. *X—XII* Vertebræ. *XIII* Hyoid Bone. 1—3. Turbinated Bones. 4. Soft Palate with Uvula. 5. Opening of the Eustachian Tube. 6. Mouth. 7. Tongue, 8. Larynx. 9. Windpipe. 10. Œsophagus. 11. Thyroid gland. 12. Epiglottis. 13. 14. Muscles of the Neck. 15. Skin.

the optic nerve passes into the brain leads into the cavity of the skull.

In front, in the inner corner the cavity of the eye is connected with the nasal cavity by the thin lacrymal duct.

The *cavity of the nose* is divided by a partition, partly bony, partly cartilaginous into a right half and into a left half; both halves are open in front and behind. The continuation of the nasal cavity behind is the choanae, (pharynx.) into which the oral cavity also leads.

The oral cavity (fig. 3) is above divided from the nasal cavity by *the palate*, of which the anterior bony part, the *hard palate* is distinguished from the posterior moveable portion, called the *soft palate*. The floor of the oral cavity is formed of tissues, which enclose the *hyoid bone*. The teeth project from the upper jaw and from the lower jaw; an adult person has sixteen teeth above and sixteen below, making thirty two altogether. There are in each jaw in front four incisors, on each side of which we find an eyetooth and five jaw-teeth. The hindmost jaw-teeth, which usually appear only after the sixteenth year are called wisdom teeth. In every tooth we distinguish the visible *crown of the tooth*, whose most important part is the hard enamel, from the root of the tooth, which is firmly fixed in the jaw. The connection between the root and the crown is called the neck of the tooth.

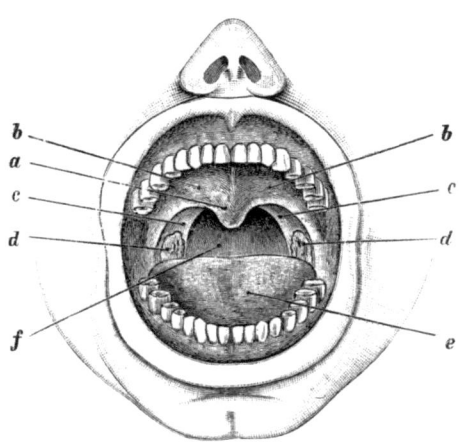

Fig. 3. *Structure of the Mouth.*
a. Uvula. *b.* Anterior palatine Arch. *c.* Posterior Palatine Arch. *d.* Tonsils. *e.* Tongue. *f.* Pharynx.

The tooth contains in its interior the soft tooth-pulp, which is traversed by bloodvessels and sensitive nerves. Behind the teeth is the tongue whose hindmost part with the soft palate bounds the narrowest spot in the cavity of the mouth. We notice at the back of the oral cavity, when the tongue is pressed down the uvula hanging down from the centre of the soft palate; at the two sides the anterior and posterior arches of the palate and the *tonsils* between the arches of the palate on each side. Under the tonsils lie two bluish transparent salivary glands; two other salivary glands are on each side of the lower edge of the lower jaw and in front of the exterior portion of this bone near the ear. The clear saliva, which is secreted by these six glands is mixed with the phlegm to be found on the mucous membrane of the cavity of the mouth.

§ 9. The Trunk; the cavities of the Trunk. The trunk finds its principal support in the *spinal column*; (also called *back bone*.) this runs from the head to the pelvis and is composed of 24 separate vertebrae; namely: seven cervical, twelve dorsal and five lumbar vertebrae. At its lower end the spinal column merges in the back of the bony pelvis, which is called the „Os sacrum". In each vertebra we distinguish in front the vertebral aperture, enclosed by the vertebral arch; and several bony projections; those projecting backwards may be externally felt in the middle line of the neck and of the back. The vertebral cavities of the vertebrae lie close above one another and form together with the cavity of the „sacrum" the tubelike vertebral canal, which is connected through the occipital aperture with the cavity of the skull and encloses the spinal cord.

From the twelve dorsal vertebrae twelve ribs, curved like a bow branch off on each side; there are therefore 24 ribs altogether; they run in a more or less sloping direction from back to front. The seven upper ribs on each side are called the true ribs, the five lower the false ribs. The ten upper rips are connected in front by cartilaginous continuations (costal cartilage) with the breastbone. This is a flat bone which runs downwards from the neck in front the middle line of the body. At its upper end are joined on both sides the two *collarbones*, which run to the shoulders.

The *pit of the stomach* or *cardiac region* is bounded upwards by the lower end of the breast bone and by the cartilage of the lower ribs which tend upwards to meet it.

The so called *Thorax* which is formed by the 24 ribs, the spinal column and the breast-bone enclose the *cavity of the chest*; (§§ 12—16). Below this lies the *abdominal cavity* (§ 18 sqq.) bounded underneath by the pelvis, behind by the lumbar vertebrae and elsewhere by tissues and separated from the thorax by a moveable partition, which consists o fa thin layer of muscles, called the *Diaphragm*. The pelvis is formed by the „*Sacrum*" and the two hip-bones; the latter are joined in front by a cartilage. On the exterior side of the hip-bones is a semi-circular hollow for the upper end of the upper femoral bone which is called the joint-pan; the part of the thigh-bone below that hollow is called the sitting-bone. The lowest part of the abdominal cavity enclosed by the pelvis is called the pelvic cavity.

§ 10. **The Upper Limbs.** In the upper limbs, the arms we distinguish the upper arm, the lower (or fore-arm) and the hand. They are connected with the trunk by the shoulders.

The bony frame of each *shoulder* is formed at the back by the shoulder-blade, a flat triangular bone lying in the back plane of the trunk; in front by the collar-bone, a ∞ like spiral tube-like bone, which runs on the lower edge of the neck almost horizontally to the breast-bone and at the sides the upper end of the upper arm-bone. This is called the *upper-armhead* and it posseses a hemi-spheroidal arched joint plane which with a glenoid cavity placed at the outer side of the shoulder-blade forms the *shoulder-joint*. Below this we find the *armpit* between the trunk and the upper arm. The bony frame of the lower arm consists of the *radius*, situated on the same side as the thumb and the ulna placed on the same side as the little finger; the hookshaped upper end of the ulna projects at the back of the elbow-joint. The radius can be moved round the ulna and thus makes possible the rotations of the hand, which follow its movements.

In the hand we distinguish the wrist, the middle hand and the fingers. The bony portion of the wrist is formed by two rows of small bones, the eight bones of the wrist, the upper row of which combines with the lower end of the radius and of the ulna to form the *joint of the hand.* In the middle hand we distinguish the *back of the hand* from the *hollow of the hand;* the latter is bounded on its side by the *ball of the thumb* and the *ball of the little finger*.

The mobility of the *fingers* is effected partly by small handmuscles situated in the middle hand, partly by the muscles of the lower arm, whose long string-shaped sinews stretch through the wrist and middle-hand as far as the finger-bones.

§ 11. **The Lower Limbs.** The *lower limbs* or *legs* begin at the *hips* and divide into upper and lower *thigh* and *foot.* The bony portion of each *upper thigh* is the *thigh-bone*, the strongest and longest bone in the human body. Its ball-shaped enlargement at the upper end forms with the glenoid cavity (§ 9) in the hip-bone the *thigh-joint*. The lower thigh, (leg) the fleshy backpart of which is called the *calf of the leg* possesses two bones, viz.: the shin-bone on the inner side and the thinner fibula on the outer side. The upper end of the shin-bone joins with the lower end of the upper thigh in the *kneejoint*, in the formation of which the flat *kneecap*, lying in front of the two bones and connected with them by strong ligaments also takes part. The back portion of the kneejoint is called the *ham*.

The two bones of the lower thigh thicken at their lower end into the inner and outer *ankle* (joint) and form with the *talus* the *joint of the foot (astralagus)*. The latter is one of the seven bones of the *tarsus*, of which the *heel bone* (oscalcis) is the most important.

The *tarsus*, the *middle foot* and the *toes* form the foot, which is again divided into the *back of the foot* (the instep) and the *sole*. In a standing position the foot rests on the heel — formed by the heeljoint — and on the balls of the big and little toes, so that the outer edge of the foot touches the ground. The heeljoint and the balls possess as fulcrum of the foot a very thick skin; that part of the sole lying between them is somewhat arched upwards and is called the *arch of the foot*. In some persons the latter has sunk so much that in standing the foot touches the ground with the whole sole and with the inner edge of the foot. A foot misshaped in that manner is called a *flat foot*. The strong sinew, which stretches like a stringlike extension of the muscles of the calf of the leg to the posterior end of the heelbone is known by the name of *The tendon of Achilles*.

§ 12. **The viscera of the thorax.** (Fig. 4.) The tissues enclosed in the large cavities of the trunk are called viscera. In the cavity of the chest lie — as *viscera of the chest* — the two lungs and the heart.

§ 13. **The Lungs and Breathing.** The lungs, of which the right is composed of three, the left of two super-imposed lobes contain like a sponge numberless very small cavities, which are called vesicles of the lungs.

From the vesicles proceed thin elastic tubes, which join in wider tubes and finally open into the large branches of the windpipe, one branch of which leads to each of the five lobes of the lungs. Two wide tubes, one of which receives the three branches of the right lung, the other the two branches of the left lung join together as the *windpipe.* (Fig. 5.)

The latter runs into the middle line of the neck and in

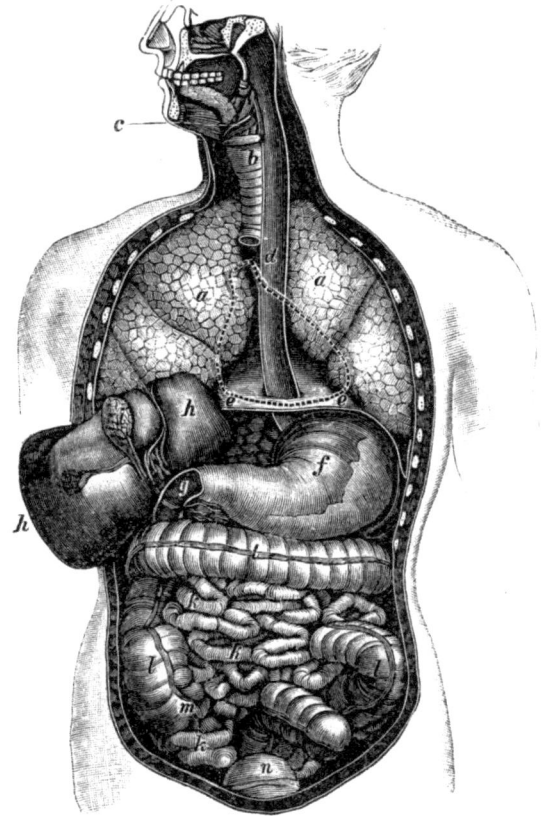

Fig. 4. *Thoracic and abdominal viscera in man.*
a. Lungs. *b.* Windpipe. *c.* Larynx. *d.* Œsophagus. *e.* Diaphragm. *f.* Stomach. *g.* Duodenum. *h.* Liver. *i.* Gallbladder. *k.* Small intestine. *l.* Large intestine. *m.* Coecum. *n.* Urinary bladder. The dotted line schows the contour (outline) of the heart, which for the sake of clearness must be considered to have been taken out. (remored.)

its upper end passes into the Larynx, which opens into the fauces and thus is connected with the outer air through the openings of the mouth and the nose. The outer surface of the lungs is covered by a thin membrane, the *pleura pulmonaris*; the interior of the chest is lined with the *pleura* (costalis).

By the uninterrupted activity of the lungs, called breathing, the air, which man requires to live, is introduced into the body. We distinguish between *inspiration* and *expiration*; in inspiration the air from without passes through the windpipe and its branches into the expanding lung-vesicles, at which action the lungs are inflated like a bellows; while in expiration the used-up air (cf. § 16 and 21) is driven out from the lung-vesicles, which process makes the expanded lungs sink down again. To inspiration and expiration correspond the regular breathing motions of the chest, which are perceptible as expansion and contraction as well as rising and falling. The air expired is warmer than the air which we inhale; it contains less oxygen than the latter, but is richer in carbonic acid and moisture; that the former contains more water can be shown, that cold objects, for instance mirrors become dulled when breathed upon, and also, that the breath, issuing from the mouth changes in cold weather into visible vapour. The number of respirations of an adult person is from 16 to 18 in a minute, but this is increased in rapid walking or running, in ascending stairs or mountains and also in several illnesses. Children when at rest and in good health also breathe more frequently.

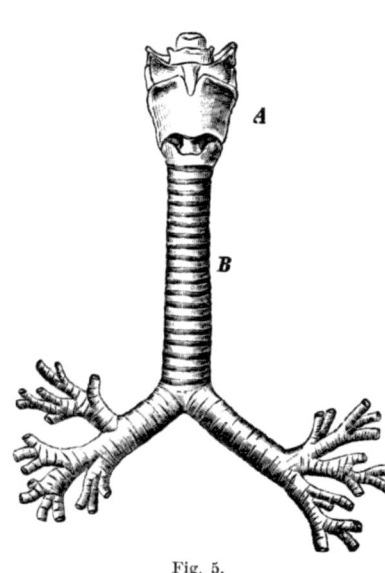

Fig. 5.
Larynx *A* and Windpipe *B* with its branches.

§ 14. **The Larynx; the voice and speech.** During the expiration tones can be produced at will in the larynx, which constitute the *voice*. The larynx, whose cartilaginous walls can be felt in the centre of the throat, contains in its interior the two vocal cords, extending close to each other from front to back. When at rest these are relaxed and lie so far apart, that a large opening between them allows free passage to the air which we breathe; but by means of small muscles in the larynx they can be extended and brought nearer to one another. The exhaled air makes them then vibrate and thus produces according to the tension of the cords higher or lower tones, which we observe in speaking and screaming, but most clearly in singing. With the aid of the tongue, the palate, the teeth an the lips we can perfect our voice to *speech*.

§ 15. The Blood; the bloodvessels; the heart and the circulation of the Blood. A part of the inhaled air mixes itself inside the lungs with the blood, which courses through the body during life in unceasing circulation. The blood is red and viscous; it consists of the colourless *blood fluid* (plasma) and innumerable little *blood corpuscles*. (Fig. 6.) By far the greater part of these are shaped like a coin and a yellow reddish colour (red blood corpuscles); a smaller number are round and colourless (white blood corpuscles). Outside the body the blood generally coagulates, as a gelatinous mass and the *bloodwater* (serum) separate from each other.

The blood is to be found partly in the *heart*, partly in conduit-like *bloodvessels*. The larger ones have elastic sides (Adern); they are divided into *arteries*, in which the blood flows from the heart into the other parts of the body, and *veins*, which bring back the blood from the body to the heart.

The *Heart* (Fig. 7), surrounded by a skin-like substance, the *pericardium* — as in a sack — lies in the front part of the left half of the thorax. It has about the size of the fist of the man, to whom it belongs, and in shape it resembles a cone whose base lies behind the middle part of the breast bone, and whose apex touches the front wall of the chest in the interval between the 5th and 6th left ribs at a distance of a hands-breadth from the lower third of the breast-bone. While the anterior wall of the heart lies close to the wall of the chest for the most part, the posterior wall and a portion of the upper and outer edges is covered by the left lung. The heart consists of muscular masses and encloses a cavity which is divided into four sections by one partition wall running vertically and another running diagonally. The two upper sections lying close to the base are called the right and left auricle; the two lower, which lie nearer to the apex are called the right and left *ventricle*. Each auricle is connected with its corresponding ventricle by an opening of the diagonal partition wall.

From the left ventricle of the heart comes out the *great artery of the body*, or *aorta*. This at first runs somewhat upwards, then makes a bend backwards to the spinal column, then from there downward to the pelvic cavity, where it divides into two „*Adern*" (arteries) for the two lower limbs. At the

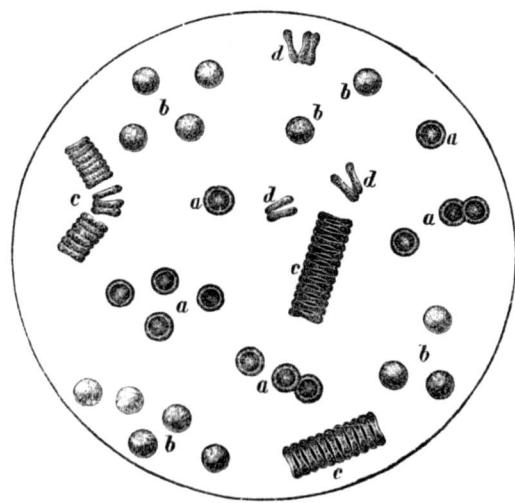

Fig. 6. *Blood corpuscles, greatly enlarged.*

a. Red; *b.* white, blood-corpuscles; *c.* red blood-corpuscles, lying besides each other, like a roll of gold; *d.* dito, seen singly laterally.

bend proceed upward from the great aorta the arteries for the head, neck and the upper limbs, while the arteries for the viscera of the thorax and abdomen come out from the aorta in its downward passage. All arteries divide into branches, till finally very thin, small arteries — *capillary vessels* — only visible by the microscope result, which are spread like a dense network all over the body. Through the uniting of capillary vessels are formed the *small veins*, and from these the *larger veins* are formed. The latter finally unite in the two great *venae cavae*, of which the upper brings back the blood from the head, neck and upper limbs and the lower the blood from the other parts of the body and pour it into the right auricle of the heart. The portion of the circulation, which we described thus far, that between the left ventricle and the right auricle of the heart is called the *great circulation,* or the „*Koerper-Kreislauf*" (circulation in the body. Fig. 8 and 9).

From the right auricle the blood passes into the right ventricle; then it enters inside the pulmonary artery proceding from there into the *small* or *lung circulation.* The pulmonary

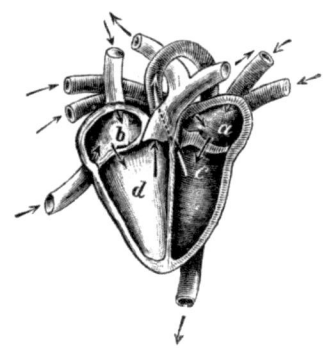

Fig. 7. *Section of the heart* (Diagramm).
a. Left auricle. *b.* Right auricle. *c.* Left ventricle. *d.* Right ventricle.

artery divides in the lungs just like the other arteries of the body into gradually smaller branches; the capillary vessels of the lungs unite and form the pulmonary veins, by which the blood is brought back to the left auricle and thus into the great circulation.

§ 16. Relations of the circulation of the blood to respiration. The circulation of the blood is effected by the contractions of the heart; these take place in an adult person about 72 times in a minute, in old age less frequently, more frequently in children, and they affect in regular alternation the auricles and the ventricles. As soon as the ventricles contract, the bood flows from them, as from a squeezed indiarubber ball into the arteries; at the same time the auricles expand and as it were suck in the blood from the bloodvessels. As soon as the auricles then contract, the blood taken up by them flows into the ventricles and expands them.

As soon as the auricles expand the apertures between them and the ventricles are closed by valve-like arrangements, so that the blood which has already passed into the ventricles cannot flow back again. Other valves prevent a reflux of the blood from the great body artery and from the pulmonary artery into the ventricles of the heart. By some diseases the valves are so changed in their shape than they are no longer capable of closing. Such *defects in the valves of the heart* may lead to disturbances in the circulation, since the blood on the expansion of the ventricles and the auricles partly flows back into them, expands them immoderately and blocks the veins.

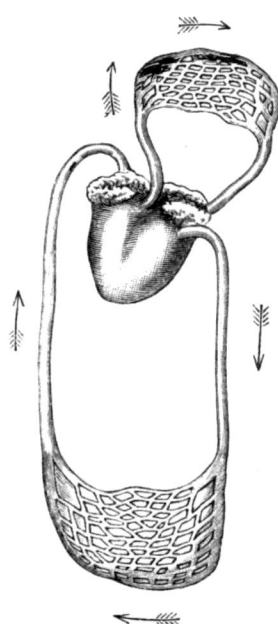

Fig. 9. *Circulation.*

Each contraction of the heart occasions a gentle motion of the chest, especially at the apex of the heart; this is the heart-beat, which is externally visible and can be felt in many men. From the influx of the blood, expanding the arteries results the beating of the pulse, which may be felt by gentle pressure of the fingertips in the superficial arteries, for instance in the radial artery inside the radius and close above the wrist. The strength and frequency of the beating of the pulse is altered in consequence of mental excitements and in many sicknesses, especially in cases of fever an increase in the number of pulse beats is usually observed.

During the circulation a change takes place in the colour of the blood, which is connected with the respiration. A part of the oxygen, contained in the inhaled air (cf. § 34) is taken up into the blood by the capillary vessels of the lung vesicles, which are provided with walls letting through the air, combines with the colouring matter of the blood contained in the

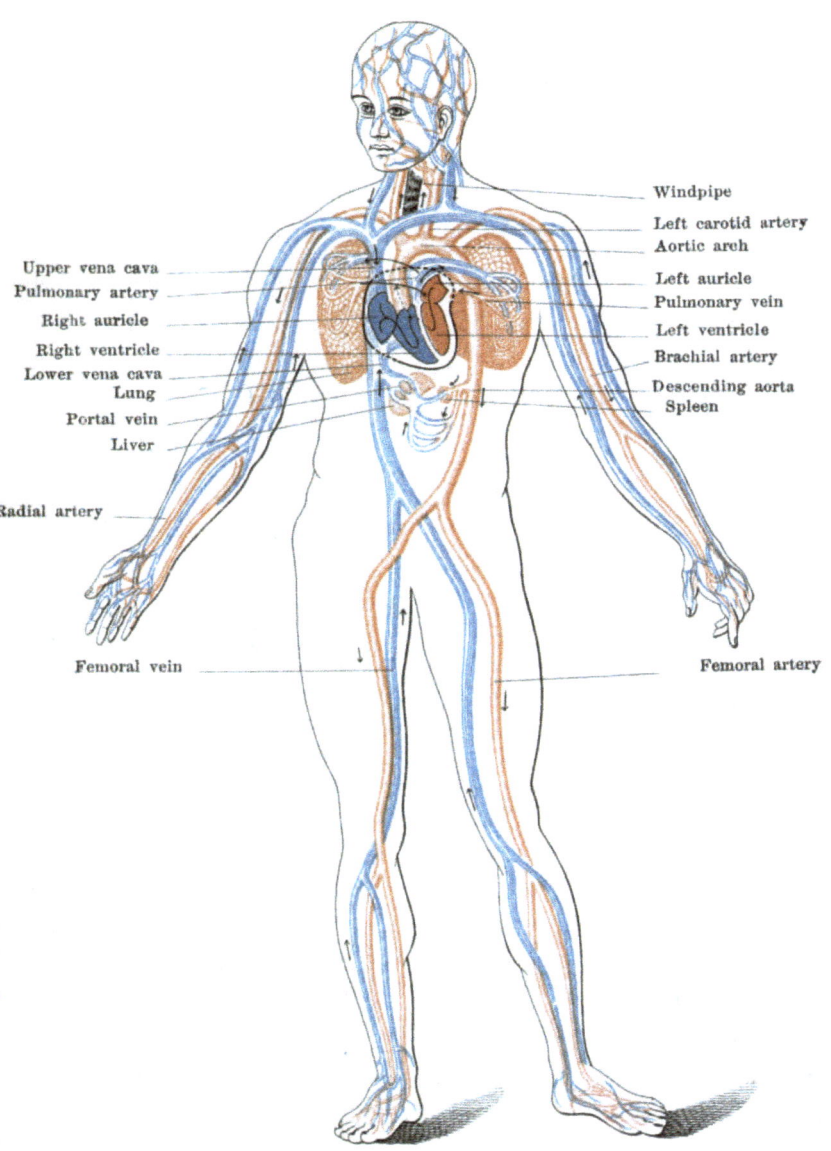

Fig. 8. *Vascular structures.*
The red vessels are arteries; the blue veins; but the pulmonary artery is coloured blue, and the pulmonary vein red, on account of the character of the blood, carried by these vessels.

red corpuscles, and thus produces the bright sclarlet red appearance of the blood. This colour remains preserved, while the blood flows through the left auricle, the left ventricle and the arteries of the body; in the capillary vessels of the great circulation the oxygen however is given up by the blood to the surrounding tissues, and an approximately equal quantity of carbonic acid is received instead, from which the blood acquires a blackish red appearance. Thus coloured the blood flows through the veins, the right auricle, ventricle and the pulmonary arteries to exchange in the lungs the carbonic acid, which it has received for fresh oxygen. The carbonic acid which is removed from the organism through exhalation is produced in the tissues of the body by a process, similar to combustion (cf. § 21),

§ 17. **Lymph, Lymph-vessels and Lymph-glands.** In addition to the arteries and veins, which convey the blood, there are still other vessels in the human body, which contain an almost colourless fluid, called *lymph*, which vessels are named lymph-vessels or absorbent vessels. Their very thin terminal branches, extending everywhere absorb their tissues from the bodily tissues and convey it into the upper *vena cava* through a great lymph vessel stretching upwards in front of the spinal column through the thorax. This vessel has a diameter of $\frac{1}{2}$ cm. Along all lymph-vessels are inserted the lymph-glands. These are varying in size from the head of a pin to a bean and contain in their interior innumerable small cells, resembling the white blood corpuscles. The lymph flowing between these cells leaves behind it as in a filter any impurities which it may have carried with it. Such impurities lead to a swelling of the lymph-glands, if they (the impurities) contained certain noxious matters absorbed from diseased bodily tissues or from wounds.

§ 18. **Viscera of the Abdomen.** (Fig. 4.) To the viscera of the abdomen belong particularly the *organs of digestion*, the *organs* for the *secretion* and *flowing off* of the urine and the *spleen*. The organs of digestion are the *stomach*, the *intestinal canal*, the liver and the *pancreas*.

§ 19. **The stomach, the oesophagus, the intestinal canal, the mesenteric and the omentum.** The stomach is a longish sack, with sides like skin; it lies crosswise immediately unter the diaphragm in midst of the abdominal cavity, the front-wall of which it touches near the cardiac region, or pit of the stomach. The more spacious part of the stomach on the left side is narrowing above and at the back to the *œsophagus;* this forms the connection between the cavity of the mouth and the stomach; it is a sack of about the thickness of a finger with an elastic side in front of the spinal column, at the neck behind the windpipe, in the thorax between the great bloodvessels downwards to the diaphragm and penetrating this latter opens into the stomach. In its part to the right the stomach narrows like a funnel, until it continues behind into the bowels. The place of transition which sometimes is compressed (constricted or gripped together) so firmly by a muscle surrounding it like a ring, that the cavity of the stomach is shut off from the interior of the bowels as if by a valve, — is called the *pylorus.*

The intestinal canal is formed like a sack with membranous walls, whose length is about six times that of the human body. We distinguish in the bowels the narrower *small intestines* from the wider *large intestine* (commonly called *great gut*). The narrow intestines, whose uppermost part, bounding on the stomach and about twelve fingers in length is called the *duodenum* fills with its folds the greater part of the cavity of the abdomen. In the lower part of the abdomen, to the right just above the hip-bone it opens into the large intestines, the first part of which lying immediately below the soft covering of the abdomen forms a sack shaped projection downwards, called the *caecum.* Hanging down from this is a *vermiform continuation,* an intestine, about as long as a finger and somewhat thicker than an earthworm. The caecum and the vermiform prolongation sometimes develop an inflammation which seriously threatens life; in some cases indigestible bodies e. g. cherry-stones, which accidentally got into the vermiform continuation are the cause of such an illness. From the *caecum* the large intestine proceeds first upwards, then it turns in front of the anterior wall of the stomach to the left side of the cavity of the abdomen, then descends into the pelvis and enters this, resting on the os sacrum as the *rectum,* in order finally to open outwards as the *posterior orifice.*

The by far largest part of the intestinal canals of the stomach, like most of the bowels of the abdomen is covered on the outside by a thin skin, the *peritoneum*, which also lines the inner wall of the abdomen. Between the peritoneum covering of the intestines and the walls of the abdomen there exist many connections in the shape of ligaments or folded membranes, which strengthen the bowels and hold them in position; these connections ar called the *mesentery*. In the front part of the abdominal cavity immediately behind the abdominal wall is the *omentum*, a membranous body hanging down loosely in front of the intestines like an apron. In the case of fat people the omentum is largely permeated with fat.

§ 20. **The liver, gall and Pancreas.** The *liver*, (which in fig. 4 for the sake of clearness — to show the organs, covered by it — is turned upwards in its total width) fills the upper part of the abdominal cavity on the right of the stomach below the diaphragm. It is a large organ — brownish red — composed of several lobes of rather solid substance; it possesses an arched upper and a more level lower surface. From the liver is secreted the *gall*, a bitter, yellow or brown fluid, which colours green when exposed to the air. The bile collects at first in the pear-shaped gall-bladder which coalesces with the lower surface of the liver and is then conducted into the duodenum through a fine conduit. At the same spot another fluid enters the interior of the bowels; this is the *juice* of the *pancreas*, which resembles saliva; the pancreas is a longish flat organ situated directly behind the stomach.

§ 21. **Digestion (Stoffwechsel).** The organs of digestion, as may be seen by the foregoing description consist on the one hand of a canal, beginning at the opening of the mouth, traversing the cavities of the trunk and ending at the opening of the posterior; and on the other hand of some glands whose secretions are discharged into the interior of this canal. The food and drink, which we consume are *digested* during their passage through this canal, i. e. the *nutritive substances* in them, which are necessary for the growth and preservation of the body are here extracted from the food and dissolved in order by the agency of the lymphatic vessels to be taken up into the blood-fluid, while the useless matter of the food leaves the body as excrement through the opening of the posterior.

We distinguish between the foodstuffs three groups, viz.: those containing *sugar* or *starch*; those with *albuminous foods* and the *fats* (cf. § 54); of these the starchy foods are especially digested by the saliva of the mouth and of the pancreas, the albuminous stuffs however are digested by the acid gastric juice, secreted by the small glands of the mucous membrane of the stomach. The change of the fats into a soluble form is effected by the agency of the bile.

The dissolution of the foodstuffs is aided or furthered by the diminution into smaller size of the food; this commences already in the opening of the mouth, where the teeth masticate every mouthful, which we eat. Then the food is getting swallowed by means of the movements of the tongue, the soft palate and the oesophagus muscles, situated in the pharynx into the oesophagus and into the stomach; while at the same time the epiglottis which is grown together with the base of the tongue, closes and prevents the entrance of food into the larynx and oesophagus (swallowing the wrong way). As soon as the stomach has received the food, it begins to secrete its gastric juice and by rotatory movements to mix thoroughly and to stir its contents; at the same time the pylorus closes, so that an immediate passage of the food into the bowels is not possible. Only when the digestion in the stomach is ended, which according to the condition of the food lasts from one to six hours, the pylorus allows the food, then changed to a thin pulp to pass into the bowels. Here the admixture of the bile of the pancreatic juice and of the juice of the intestines, secreted by the small glands in the mucous membrane of the bowels effect an almost complete fluidity of the (what is called) *chyme*. The fluid, thus produced, coloured yellow by the bile is by the aid of the rotatory movements in the intestines (similar to the contortions of a worm) gradually sent through the long thin intestines, assumes gradually a more and more pulpy and then a viscous character, and finally changes inside the great intestines into the still more solid excrements.

This gradual thickening of the contents of the intestines is the result of a transference of its fluid parts to the circulating lymph and blood; especially in the small intestines the lymph-vessels of the mucous membrane of the gut absorb a milky-white fluid — the chyle — which then conduct into the principal lymph-vessel and thus into the circulating blood. By the blood the chyle is carried to the cells, of which the tissue of the body is composed, and is assimilated by them in order to be used for the formation of new tissue and partly for the preservation of the old cells. The action of the individual cells which lies at the basis of all functions of life requires an unceasing consumption of the chemical matter, of which the human body is constructed. A process, similar to combustion is thereby carried out. The chemical constituents of the cell-body are by the help of the oxygen supplied by the blood converted into more simple chemical compounds, especially into carbonic acid, water and a residue corresponding to the ash of combustible bodies. Combustion and the function of cells differ in so far as the former ordinarily takes place with the production of light, the latter generally without it; but both have in common the production of heat together with the consumption of the material employed. As for the maintenance of every combustion a constant supply of combustible material is necessary, so for the continuance of the cell-activity of our body, without which life would be impossible always new cellular tissue, supplied by the chyle is indispensable.

The continual consumption and replacing of the consumed nutritive food — by the aid of the supply of oxygen and nourishment through breathing and digestion is called the assimilation of the living body.

§ 22. **The heat of the Body. Fever.** The heat produced by the cell activity is distributed by means of the blood in an almost uniform manner over the whole body. The body thus aquires *heat of its own*, which varies only some tenths of a degree during the day and in healthy man stands on an average at about 37^0 C. Any considerable increase in the temperature of the body is prevented by the fact, that a part of the heat of the body is being constantly given off to the surrounding air, from the surface of the body, 2^d with the exhaled air, 3^d with the secretions. This giving off of heat is sometimes increased by perspiration, as the evaporation of the moisture, produced on the surface of the skin acts as a withdrawer of heat. In summer, when the air is so warm, that the body cannot cool itself sufficiently by giving off of heat from its surface, the glands of the skin give out more perspiration than at the other seasons of the year. An immoderate cooling of the body is prevented by the clothing which protects in our climate the surface of the skin from the effects of the colder air.

By illness the temperature of the body may be increased; temporarily also by very great activity of the muscles (§ 193 and § 185). Its increase to 41.5 and higher usually brings about the death of man. On severe exhaustion and in similar circumstances the temperature sometimes sinks to 36^0 C., and occasionally even lower; after death the cessation of the activity of the cells causes a rapid cooling of the body.

§ 23. **Urine; the Kidneys** and **the Urinary canals.** At the decomposition of the constituents of the body connected with the activity of the cells certain waste matter (§ 21) remains behind, which at once passes into the blood — namely carbonic acid, water and so-called ashes. A part of the water escapes with the carbonic acid into the exhaled air; the rest of the water, not required in the body leaves the organism in the form of *sweat* (cf. § 6) and of *urine* together with certain ash substances to which it serves as a means of solution.

The urine of a healthy person is a clear fluid, coloured sometimes lighter yellow, sometimes darker yellow or reddish yellow according to the proportion of water which it contains. In the open air it soon putrifies, owing to the formation of ammonia, at the same time it gets muddy. As in cases of bad health the urine of the patient not infrequently shows traces of cellular and other matter also sugar or dissolved albumin, its chemical or microscopical examination often discloses to the physician the nature of the illness.

The urine is secreted through the two kidneys, which are grayish or brownish-red bean-shaped glands, about 10 to 15 cm long; which lie, embedded in rich fatty tissues on both sides of the lumbar vertebræ next to the posterior wall of the abdominal cavity. From the hollow of each kidney, called the *pelvis of the kidney* leads the urinary duct — similar to an india-rubber tube to the bladder, which lies in the pelvic cavity in front of the rectum. From the bladder the urine is emptied externally from time to time.

§ 24. **The Spleen.** Besides the organs of digestion and the urinary organs there is also in the abdominal cavity the *spleen*, a long flat organ of bluish-red colour of rather strong tissue, which plays a part in the formation of blood. The spleen lies on the left of the stomach between the diaphragm and the left kidney; it is usually completely covered by the lower ribs, but grows in some cases of illness to such a size, that its edge can be felt through the covering of the abdomen on the left side below the last ribs.

§ 25. The action of the nerves. The Brain, and the spinal marrow. While the circulation of the blood, breathing and digestion are accomplished in the living organism regularly and unconsciously without being influenced by the will, there are other functions in the life of the human body, which require the presence of consciousness and to some degree re-

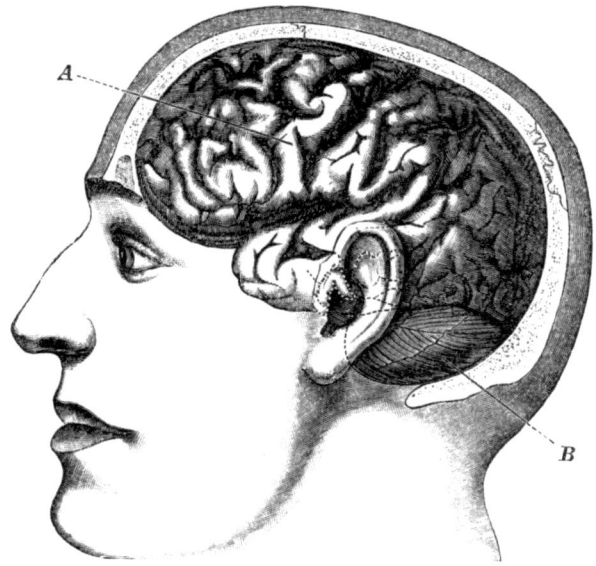

Fig. 10. *Position of the Brain.*
A. The great brain. B. The little brain.

present the activity of the will. These are the *sensations*, by means of which we become conscious of the objects and events around us and a large part of the *movements*.

The capacity for *sensation* and for voluntary movement is combined with the possession of *nerves* and with the principal organs, that belong to them. The brain and the spinal marrow form the centre of the activity of the nerves.

The *brain* (Fig. 10) forms the contents of the cavity of the skull; it is surrounded by several, partly hard, partly tender membranes and consists of a mass of soft tissues, traversed by many bloodvessels which for the most part are narrow and of thin sides. We distinguish in the brain-mass the superficial thin grayish coloured *cortex* from the more extensive *white mass* (the kernel). The latter contains in its interior several gray-coloured patches and several cavities connected with each other, containing a watery fluid. The whole organ is separated by a cross-fissure into an anterior, larger principal part called the *great brain* and a smaller part, the *little brain*, occupying the posterior lower portion of the cavity of the skull. A longitudinal fissure divides the great brain and the small brain into right and left halves. Besides we distinguish in the brain so-called *lobes*, which are named according to their position frontal — middle — temporal and occiput-lobes; and in each lobe we distinguish some convolutions. Between the lobes and convolutions there are to be found on the surface of the brain some irregular peculiarly-curved furrows, which however penetrate less deeply into the mass of organs than the great longitudinal and lateral fissures.

The *spinal marrow* fills the vertebral canal; like the brain it is surrounded by membranes, is of a cylindrical shape and is composed of a soft tissue, white outside and gray inside. With its upper end, the so-called prolonged spinal marrow enters the cavity of the skull to change here immediately to the brain; the cavities of the brain are continued into the thin canal of the spinal marrow which traverses the latter from top to bottom.

In the gray mass of the brain and of the spinal marrow are innumerable structures only visible through the microscope, the so-called *ganglion-cells*. From the peculiar edges of these cells proceed very thin *nerve filaments* which at a short distance unite in white bundles, called *nerve-fibres*. The nerve-fibres compose the white mass of the brain of the spinal marrow; they cross each other on many places in the brain, but run lengthwise through the spinal marrow, close to one onother, like bundles of string. Out of the nerve-fibres are formed the *nerves*, which leave the brain and spinal marrow as white, strong strings of about the thickness of a knitting needle to a quill-pen, then again split into single bundles and filaments owing to repeated divisions and bifurcation, and finally terminate in the most varions parts of the body as very minute structures, only visible through the microscope.

The ganglion-cells of the brain are the seat of consciousness; in them our conceptions are formed, and in them the will has its origin, which governs our actions. The nerves undertake the transmission between the ganglion-cells (whence they proceed) and the various parts of the body, which receive the sensations and execute the actions that are directed by the will. The destruction of certain portions of the brain, which may occur in consequence of external injuries or as the result of bleeding from bursting brain-vessels (apoplexy of the brain) causes the loss of some capacities of certain definite conceptions or movements according to the place of injury, owing to the interruption of the nerve fibres, or the annihilation of the ganglion-cells. Thus after the destruction of a certain convolution in the left frontal lobe of the great brain a man loses the capacity of forming words, injuries to other neighbouring parts of the brain result in palsy of the limbs; the faculties of seeing or hearing may also be lost by injury to certain parts of the brain. In a similar manner the functions of certain portions of the body will be made impossible by the severance of the nerve connecting it with the brain. Thus the cutting of an optic nerve causes the immediate blindness of the eye connected with that nerve.

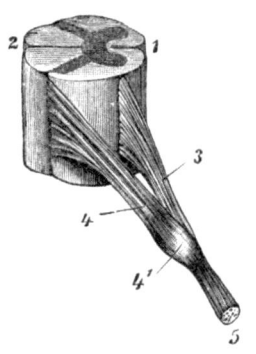

Fig. 11. *The Origin of a spinal-marrow nerve.*
1 2 Spinal column. *3 4* Roots of the nerve. *5* Nerve.

Of the single nerves the most important are the twelve pairs of *cerebral nerves* which leave the cavity of the skull through certain apertures in its osseous wall. Some of them, as for instance the nerves of sight, hearing and taste convey to the brain sense-perceptions; others are *motor nerves*, like the nerves of the eye-muscles, the two nerves of the muscles of the face, and the two nerves of the tongue.

From the spinal marrow proceed thirty pairs of *spinal nerves;* each of these has an anterior and a posterior root (Fig. 11); through the posterior roots proceed those nerve-filaments which convey *sensations* to the spinal cord and to the brain; the anterior root is composed of those nerve-filaments, running from the spinal cord and from the brain to the organs of movement. Through the injury or destruction of the posterior root of a spinal cord nerve certain portions of the body lose their sensibility, while similar lesions in the region of the anterior root result in the paralysis of certain definite muscles.

§ 26. **The organs of sense.** For the reception of the sensations, produced by external impressions and conveyed by the nerves to the brain the body possesses special sense-organs of sight, hearing, taste, smell and touch.

§ 27. **The sense of sight. The eyes.** The *two eyes* are the organs of the sense of sight. We distinguish in each eye the eyeball and its auxiliary and protective contrivances.

The two *eyeballs* (Fig. 12) lie in the cavities of the eyes, embedded in soft fatty tissue, and possess about the size (circumference) and shape of large cherries. They are joined to the brain by the two optic nerves, each of which passes from the cavity of the skull through an aperture (Fig. 8) into the cavity of the eye (orbit) and enters the posterior wall of the eye to dissolve there in nerve-filaments. We distinguish in each eyeball a firm coating, similar to the rind of a fruit and a gelatinous transparent contents, called the *vitreous body*. The coating consists of three layers. The outer layer is formed by the porcelain-white and firmly fixed *hard skin* (sclerotic) and is a protective covering for the inner parts of the eye-ball. A part of its anterior is known as the „White of the eye". The middle layer is the *choroid*, a tender tissue,

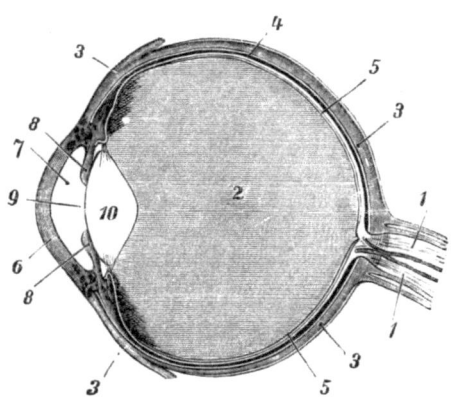

Fig. 12. *Section of the eye-ball* (enlarged).

1. Optic nerve. *2.* Vitreous body. *3.* Sclerotic. *4.* Choroid. *5.* Retina. *6.* Cornea. *7.* Anterior chamber. *8.* Iris. *9.* Pupil. *10.* Crystalline lens.

coloured black on its inner surface, in which the bloodvessels, running to the eyeball branch out. The inner layer is the *retina*, a fine very soft network of the filaments of the optic nerve. On the anterior surface of the sclerotic is a circular slightly convex transparent division, the *cornea* through which the light falls into the interior of the eye, as through a window. The part of the choroid, lying behind does not touch the cornea, but is stretched like a curtain between the space formed by its convexity — the *anterior chamber* — and the interior of the eye. This part of the choroid is called the *iris* because it is differently coloured in different persons. According to its colour we speak of gray, blue, brown or black eyes. The iris has in its centre a round aperture, the pupil of the eye, which appears as the „black in the eye". According as the pupil dilates or contracts, it allows more or less light to fall into the interior of the eye. The iris therefore represents a contrivance, which is able to soften or to lessen a too strong light by contraction of the pupil. Behind the pupil, immediately in front of the vitreous body lies the *crystalline lens*, a body formed of transparent, strong tissue, which is curved in front and behind like a magnifying-glass. The crystalline lens unites the rays of light, passing through the cornea and the pupil on the background of the eye into an image, which is received (retained) by the retina.

By the ordinary convexity of the lens only rays of light falling parallel into the eye are combined on the back ground of the eye, while rays entering obliquely only unite behind the back of the eye. As only rays, coming from an immensely great distance strike the eye in parallel lines, the lens possesses the faculty of increasing its convexity by muscular activity so as to focus also the rays coming obliquely from a near distance on the background of the eye.

There are however eyes of such a small length diameter, that the lens must increase its convexity in order to focus even parallel rays on the retina, and cannot focus oblique rays at all on the back of the eye, so that the image, produced on the retina is rendered indistinct. We call such eyes *oversighted.* Their power of vision can be improved by an artificial lens, which supplements the action of the crystalline lens in the shape of a double-convex eyeglass placed before the eye. Other eyes, which are constructed with such a long diameter that the focussing of the parallel rays takes place already before they reach the back of the eye are only able to perceive clearly near images, as rays coming from near objects strike the eye obliquely and are therefore focussed at a greater distance from the lens than parallel rays. We call such eyes near-sighted, and their visual capacity is improved by the use of eye-glasses, which are grounded double concave and which scatter the rays of light before they can reach the eye.

With higher age the power of the lens of focussing itself for rays coming from near gradually decreases. The near-point of sight i. e. the smallest distance at which the eye can see an object plainly, recedes more and more; the eye can — relatively speaking — only perceive clearly very distant objects; it becomes *longsighted.* In popular „parlance" this term is also used — not quite appropriately — for oversighted eyes.

A grayish dimness of the lens, arising from injury to the eye or from sickness and particularly from very old age diminishes or destroys the visual power of the eye and is called *cataract.* By a removal — through an operation — of the lens, which has become opacous (opaque) persons attacked by star can again recover their eye-sight; but they must afterwards constantly wear highly convex spectacles instead of the removed lens.

The eyeballs can be moved in several directions by the muscles, lying with them in the cavity of the eyes and therefore can be directed towards different objects in quick succession. A wider vision around is made possible by the movements of the head. As soon as both eyes at the same moment are directed towards a near object, they perceive it from different sides, and thus the form of the object perceived can easier be imaged. When looking straight ahead the muscles of the eyes are in a state of counteraction; i. e. the action of the muscles on the inner-side of the eyeball is counterbalanced by the action by those acting from outside. A disturbance of this counterpoise, which may be due to various causes produces *squinting.* If for instance the outer muscle of the eye is in a state of weakness, or if the inner muscle is shortened, the direction of the affected eye will be more inside, which causes squinting inward.

By certain *protective arrangements* the eyes are preserved

from external injuries. The *eyelids* especially protect the eyeballs from the intrusion of foreign bodies (for instance *insects*) and prevent by means of the thin hairs (hanging) on their edges (eyelashes) dust or other foreign bodies getting into the eye. The surface of the lids, next to the eye is covered by a membrane, the so called *conjunctiva*, which is continued over the anterior surface of the eyeball.

The *lachrymal fluid* serves for the removal of particles of dust, which notwithstanding the protection of the eyelids and eyelashes have penetrated into the space between the lids and the eyeball, called the conjunctiva sack.

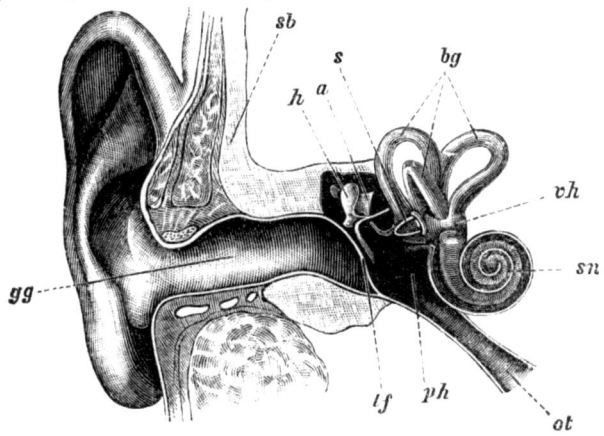

Fig. 13. Section of the Ear.

gg. Outer auditory canal. *tf.* Tympanum. *ph.* Tympanic cavity. *ot.* Eustachian Tube. *h.* Malleus. *a.* Incus. *s.* Stapes. *bg.* Semi-circular Canals. *vh.* Vestibule. *sp.* Cochlea. *sb.* Temporal bone.

The fluid is secreted by the *lachrymal glands*, which are also lying in the cavities of the eyes and gets into the conjunctiva sack whence it ordinarily flows into through the lachrymal duct into the cavity of the nose. In weeping an increased secretion of the lachrymal fluid takes place. Also when the conjunctiva becomes red from inflammation of the eye or when it swells up, or discharges freely „pus" and matter, a „running of the eyes" takes place, as the thin apertures, which lead to the lachrymal duct become more or less impassable, by which the flowing off of the lachrymal fluid into the nose is prevented.

§ 28. The sense of Hearing. The Ears. The two ears are the organs of the sense of hearing. (Fig. 13.)

By their intervention the *sound-vibrations* become perceptible. We distinguish in each ear a sound-receiving part, the *external ear*, a sound-conducting part, the *middle ear*, and a sound-perceiving part, the *inner ear*.

The outer ear consists of the *ear-shell*, which is formed of cartilage; and of the *outer auditory* which leads into the skull. The *ear-wax* is secreted by fine glands, opening into the surface of the outer auditory. On the boundary between the outer auditory and the middle ear is stretched a thin, elastic membrane, the ear-drum (tympanum). The middle ear consists of the *tympanic cavity*, the *ear-trumpet* (Eustachian canal) and the *auditory bones*. The tympanic cavity is a small cavity, filled with air and which communicates with the nasal portion of the pharynx by a thin tube, covered with a mucous membrane. (The Eustachian canal.) The auditory bones, which according to their shape are called malleus, incus and stapes are joined together by tender ligaments. The *inner ear* or labyrinth is composed of the three semi-circular canals, the vestibule and the cochlea and represents a cavity which is filled with fluid. The end of the auditory nerve, which runs through a canal in the bone of the skull from the brain to the ear divides in the cochlea into many small filaments, lying close together like the keys of a piano.

The soundwaves are received by the shell of the ear and by the auditory canal and conveyed thence to the tympanum, which thereby is made to vibrate. The vibrations are transmitted by means of the auditory bones and set into motion the fluid of the inner ear, whereby the nerve filaments are getting stimulated and the sound sensations are conveyed to the brain.

The tympanum is endangered by a too loud sound, as it can be burst by violent sound-vibrations owing to its (the tympanum's) tender quality. This danger is however obviated in the following manner; the sound-waves by the connection, maintained through the ear-trumpet between the tympanic cavity and the openings of the mouth and of the nose, reach the tympanum not only from the outer ear, but also from the middle ear and thus mutually weaken each other. To facilitate this countereffect between the sound-waves it is advisable to open the mouth during very loud noises (cannonshot, explosions, etc.) to allow the air the widest possible passage to the ear-trumpet. (Eustachian canal.)

§ 29. Taste; Smell; Touch. The *sensations of taste* are produced by substances, which are soluble in the fluid of the mouth, — the saliva —. They are communicated to the brain by means of the *gustatory nerves*, whose end fibres are enclosed in the small warts — papillae, — which are visible on the surface of the tongue.

The *sensations of smell* are received by the two *olfactory nerves*, which run from the brain to the sides of the cavity of the nose and whose end fibrils are in the mucous membrane of the nose only volatile substances, which are conducted by the air to the moist mucous membrane of the nose can be perceived by the sense of smell.

The sensations of touch are brought about through the *sensory nerves,* which terminate in the under-skin. An irritation of the ends of the sensory sometimes produces pain, sometimes a sensation of cold or heat; we can also perceive by means of these nerves every contact of the skin and estimate every pressure according to its strength. We therefore speak of *sensations of pain,* of *temperature,* of *contact* and of *pressure.* We estimate the *weight of an object* on the one hand by the effort, which the muscles make in lifting it, and on the other hand by the sensation of pressure which it causes.

§ 30. Sleep. The brain, constantly occupied by a great number of sense perceptions occasionally requires rest and recreation, which it gets by *sleep.* During sleep breathing, the circulation of the blood and digestion pursue their course without interruption, while consciousness disappears and the voluntary muscles cease their activity. At the same time the ultimate products of the process of food-assimilation, resulting from the work of the body when awake, and which cause a feeling of weariness, are removed from the organs by the circulating blood and by lymph; and are then carried off partly by breathing, partly through the agency of the kidneys and sweat-glands.

In healthy, quiet sleep the respirations are less frequent and deeper than in the waking state. The duration of sleep is regulated according to age. The infant sleeps upward to 20 hours daily; the growing child sleeps gradually a shorter time; in its seventh year it requires about seven hours sleep. For an adult person six to eight hours sleep are sufficient. Generally the need of sleep is regulated by the amount of work which a person has to perform; still strong persons require less sleep than weakly persons. Old people often can sleep but a short time, but they try to make good this loss by a longer time of rest in bed.

§ 31. **Propagation.** In the body of man, as in every other living creature the germs for new creatures of the same species develop themselves. When the formation of the juvenile body has progressed so far, that the individual can take an independent place in creation — with the capacity of working independently — then usually the organs for propagating and increasing the human race are fully developed. Considerations of health require, that the work of these organs should only commence, when the human being is quite grown up, fully developed in body and in the fulness of strength.

B. The necessaries of life for the individual man.

§ 32. The necessaries of man's life in general. The conditions for the preservation of the life of the individual man are not completely fulfilled by the perfect structure and healthy state of his body. The functions of his organs, without which his life is not possible presuppose the fulfillment of certain *wants* (*necessaries*), which can only be supplied by the surrounding world. Thus man requires *air* for breathing, *water* for drinking and cleansing, *food* and *provisions* to maintain the work of assimilation, *clothes* and *dwellings* to protect his individual warmth against the influence of the weather. *Light* is also an indispensable want and lastly *intellectual stimulation*, which can be the less dispensed with, the higher the stage of development is, to which man has raised himself by education and culture.

The knowledge of the best method of satisfying those requirements of life forms the chief aim of *hygienic science*.

I. The Air.

§ 33. The atmosphere and its composition. The air, which is required by men and animals for breathing surrounds the earth as atmosphere in a layer about 75 to 90 km (47—56 engl. miles) high. It consists of a mixture of several gases in the following proportions. 100 litres (gallons) of air contain about 78 gallons nitrogen, 21 l oxygen, $\frac{1}{30}$ l carbonic acid, and a variable quantity of watery vapour. Recently some more, until now unknown gaseous constituents were discovered, of which the most important is *Argon*.

§ 34. Nitrogen, oxygen and carbonic acid of the air. *Nitrogen* (called in German *Stickstoff*, i. e. choke-gas) which forms the chief mass of the air is thus named, because it cannot support life by itself. A man, placed in a space filled with nitrogene alone would choke. Nitrogen has no influence on the functions of the body.

Oxygen is indispensable, not only for human and animal life (§ 13 and 16), but also for the processes of combustion and decomposition of all substances, belonging to the animal and vegetable kingdoms. Its effect, which takes places under certain conditions and is called *oxydation* is of a purely chemical nature. It dissolves the organic substances and combines with the carbon and hydrogen, contained in them to form carbonic acid and water. In spite of the continual large consumption of oxygen its proportion in the composition of the air remains almost unchanged, as the quantities consumed are replaced by plants. For there is a perpetual exchange taking place between animal and plant life, as the carbonic acid, exhaled by men and animals is dissolved again into its elements by the plants, and produces on the one hand the carbon, necessary for the structure of the body of the plant, on the other hand the oxygen, required by men and animals for the air which they are breathing. Moreover the plants also replace the consumed oxygen of the air by decomposition of the water absorbed by their roots and leaves; the hydrogen of the water entering into chemical combination with the carbon, that was extracted from the carbonic acid.

Under the influence of electrical discharges during thunderstorms or the evaporation of water in the case of rain and dew a portion of the oxygen, contained in the air condenses itself to two thirds of the space, originally filled by it. In this way is produced a special kind of oxygen, called *ozone;* its presence in the air can be perceived by means of its peculiar smell and it possesses the power of oxydation in a still higher degree than the ordinary oxygen. The importance of ozone for the body and health was formerly considered very high; at present only a purifying influence on the air and thus merely a mediate influence on man are ascribed to it.

Carbonic acid passes constantly into the atmosphere in large quantities through all processes of combustion as well as through the breathing of men and animals. The air exhaled by an adult man during an hour contains about 22 to 23 litres of carbonic acid. Besides it is produced by all processes of putrefaction on the surface of the globe; it also escapes into the air from some springs, mines, earth-fissures and volcanoes.

Carbonic acid is a poison for men and animals. Of course,

the small quantity of it contained in the air inhaled, mixed with nitrogen and oxygen as it is can be inhaled without injury, but injurious effects manifest themselves as soon as the quantity of carbonic acid in the air increases e. g. in the neighborhood of carbon-rich springs or in the fermenting cellars of beer-breweries. The inhalation of air, which in a thousand parts contains from 1 to 5 parts carbonic acid causes discomfort, dizziness, headache and nausea; in air, which contains 30 per cent carbonic acid men die soon.

§ 35. Moisture and Heat of the air. The degree of *moisture* of the *air*, i. e. the *amount* of *water*, mixed invisibly with the atmosphere by evaporation is of importance for our well-being. Dry air withdraws water and heat from the body, whereby the skin becomes chapped and cracked, the mucous membrane of the throat dry, the voice hoarse and a feeling of thirst takes place. In moist air the water, evaporated from the surface of the body cannot evaporate sufficiently, the cooling of the skin decreases and an oppressive discomfort arises; we feel a slight increase of heat in such air as disagreable „sultriness".

The amount of water in the atmosphere is subject to considerable *variations*.

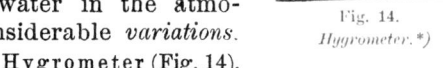

Fig. 14.
Hygrometer.*)

It is measured by the Hygrometer (Fig. 14). The simplest form of this instrument depends upon the observation, that a human hair gets longer in moist air and again shorter in dry air, or that a woody fibre gets bent in dry air and straightens again in moist air.

In places, where facilities for large evaporation of water exist, for instance on the seashore, on lakes, rivers and other expanses of water, over meadows and woods the air is usually moister than over sandy soil, dry steppes and deserts. But there is a limit, over which the air cannot absorb water. This limit is called the *saturation point* and it is indicated by

---

*) The perspective of this figure ist not quite correct; in order that it may be more easily understood.

numbers, showing, how many grammes of water in a vaporous form a cubic metre of air can hold. The height of the saturation-point depends on the heat, which the air receives, either direct from the sun, either from the surface of the earth and the living beings on it. The saturation point (according to *Fluegge*) is at a

		Saturation-point
Temperature of the air of	$-20°$ C.	1.06
,, ,, ,, ,, ,,	$-10°$ C.	2.30
,, ,, ,, ,, ,,	$\pm 0°$ C.	4.87
,, ,, ,, ,, ,,	$+10°$ C.	9.37
,, ,, ,, ,, ,,	$+20°$ C.	17.06
,, ,, ,, ,, ,,	$+30°$ C.	30.14

In consequence of this mutual relations of between the saturation-point of the atmosphere and its heat warm air is as a rule moister than cold air.

The heat of the air is measured by the *thermometer*. This is usually a thin, airless glasstube, filled partly with alcohol or mercury; its lower end widens into a spherical reservoir and its upper end is hermetically closed; it indicates changes of the temperature by rising or falling of the fluid, as alcohol or mercury are expanded by heat or contracted by cooling in a particularly easily visible manner. For the purpose of having a uniform designation of the different degrees of the temperature, the tube of the thermometer is provided with a graduated scale, for the limits of which the *boiling point* and the *freezing point* were chosen, i. e. those points, to which the alcohol or the mercury reach in the tube of the thermometer, when it is placed in the vapour of boiling water or in melting snow. The portion of the glasstube lying between these two points is divided in the *Celsius* Thermometer, which is now almost in general use in Germany into 100 equal parts, in the *Reaumur* thermometer formerly in use in Germany in 80 equal parts, and in the *Fahrenheit* thermometer, mostly used in England into 180 equal parts, called degrees. Thus an increase of heat of $10°$ Celsius is equivalent to an increase of 8 degrees Reaumur and 18 degrees Fahrenheit. By means of a similar continuation of the gradation beyond the boiling and freezing points the indication of a still higher or lower temperature is made possible. In the Celsius and Reaumur thermometers the freezing point is marked zero (0), the degrees above it are marked (+), as degrees of heat and the lower as degrees of cold (—). The freezing point of a Fahrenheit thermometer is marked 32 degrees, and the boiling point marks therefore 212 degrees. In indicating a certain temperature we use for the word degrees the abbreviation $°$ with the addition of the Initial of the thermometer used; for instance for 11 degrees heat according to a Celsius thermometer we write $+11°$ C., 14 degrees cold according to a Reaumur thermometer $-14°$ R.; the following table shows the corresponding degrees on the three scales of the 3 thermometers.

C.	R.	F.	C.	R.	F.
$-17.8°$	$-14.2°$	$0°$	$+50°$	$+40°$	$+122°$
$-10°$	$-8°$	$+14°$	$+60°$	$+48°$	$+140°$
$0°$	$0°$	$+32°$	$+70°$	$+56°$	$+158°$
$+10°$	$+8°$	$+50°$	$+80°$	$+64°$	$+176°$
$+20°$	$+16°$	$+68°$	$+90°$	$+72°$	$+194°$
$+30°$	$+24°$	$+86°$	$+100°$	$+80°$	$+212°$
$+40°$	$+32°$	$+104°$			

§ 36. **Movement of the air. Deposits.** By getting warmer the air not only increases its aequeous contents, but also expands to a larger space and thus becomes thinner. Consequently warm air is lighter than cold air, i. e. a cubic metre of thin, rarefied warm air weighs less than a cubic metre of dense, cold air. Hence warm air shows a tendency of rising, whereas cold air descends. As the layers of the atmosphere, nearest to the warm surface of earth are especially warmed, and as these layers are not of the same temperature in different parts of the globe, an interchange takes continually place between the hot and cold layers of air; these processes are the principal cause of *changes in the weather*, on the one hand the currents of air caused by this interchange become in certain conditions so strong, that we feel them as *wind;* on the other hand the originally warm air, as soon as it gets cooled becomes incapable of retaining all its water in gaseous form; a part of the latter is separated from it in the form of small watery particles and becomes visible to our eyes in the form *of fog* or *clouds*. In case of still stronger cooling they form *rain, snow* and hail, the known atmospherie *deposits*. As the heating of the air is greatest at the Equator, the cooling strongest over the Poles, the above-mentioned meteorological phaenomena are especially produced by the influence of two opposite currents of air, of which one conveys the warm air from the equator to the poles, *(the equatorial current)* whereas the other moves the cold polar air to the equator *(polar current)*. Both currents suffer certain changes in their direction in consequence of the rotation of the earth.

The human body feels the movement of the air only, if the air-current travels at a rate of at least $\frac{1}{2}$ metre in a second. The average velocity of the movement of the air (strength of the wind) is estimated at 3 metres per second. If the layer of air, nearest to the human body changes so quickly in consequence of the rapid motion of the air, that the withdrawal of heat and moisture is considerably increased, we experience a feeling of cold.

§ 37. The pressure of the air.

The pressure of the air is closely connected with its temperature and its motion. The pressure of the air is the load which the atmosphere exercises by reason of its weight. As a rule we do not feel this pressure which constantly weighs upon the surface of our body; but we can convince ourselves of its presence, if by ascending the tops of high mountains we diminish it by the layers of air, through which we have passed. As the air on account of the diminished pressure from above is less dense in the higher layers of the atmosphere, we involuntarily increase the number of respirations in order to inhale sufficient oxygen. In spite of this we do not obtain a sufficient supply of oxygen; we feel ourselves fatigued, relaxed and sleepy. Through the bursting of small blood vessels, upon the walls of which the atmospheric pressure from the outside does not correspond any longer to the pressure of the blood within bleeding at the mouth and nose occurs; we miss the usual firmness in our joints, since the ends of the bones are not pressed against one another in their sockets with the customary weight in consequence of the diminished pressure of the atmosphere. To such discomforts, which the dwellers of the lowlands freqently experience on high mountains we give the name of „*mountain-sickness*".

The pressure of the atmosphere is subject to freqent changes; on a rise of the temperature and moisture of the air it diminishes in proportion to the decrease in its weight caused thereby, and increases when the air becomes colder and more dry.

The atmospheric pressure is measured by means of the barometer (Fig. 15). Its most usual form is the quicksilver-barometer; it consists of a glasstube bent in the form of a U. In one arm of the tube, which is closed at the top and air-less, is a column of mercury, which is held in equilibrium by the weight of the atmosphere, pressing on the open end of the other arm; so that the top of the mercury-column stands higher or lower according to the greater or lesser pressure of the atmosphere. At the level of the sea the average pressure of the atmosphere can hold in equilibrium a column of mercury 760 mm high; on higher points of the surface of the earth, where the pressure of the atmosphere is less, the barometer stands lower.

Another form of barometer, the capsule- or *aneroid-barometer* is based

I. The air. 41

on the fact, that a thin metal box, which is made as „air-less" as possible, becomes compressed by an increase of the pressure of the atmosphere and expands when the pressure diminishes. The motions, thus caused in the side of the box are transmitted by a special contrivance to a dial, and by the latter are made visible and measurable on a surface provided with a graduated scale.

The variations in the atmospheric pressure are closely connected with changes in the weather. In sultry weather the pressure of the air is usually lower as for instance ordinarily before a thunderstorm; winds increase or diminish the pressure according as they bring cold or moist warm air.

§ 38. **Contamination of the air.** The air contains usually a larger or smaller quantity of impurities. Among them are the effluvia of human beings, which are especially noticeable in sleeping rooms or in densely inhabited dwellings; (cf. § 34) further, the gases, developed in many manufacturing trades, which molest us already by their disagreable smell. Considerable numbers of small bodies can be perceived as sunbeams, as soon as a ray of sunlight falls through a chink into a dark room. To these solid particles in the air belong also the dust, produced by the movement in human dwellings or the dust furnished by industrial works or the soot driven upwards into the air from chimneys or furnaces. Such contaminations of the air may not only molest our respiratory organs, but they can also become injurious to our health, particularly as such dust in the air may be a carrier of disease (cf. § 188) germs, and may even convey to us directly contagious diseases. The moist surface of the airpassages forms a protection against the intrusion of injurious dust particles into the body, and especially their manyfolded windings in the nasal cavity; thus many particles of dust remain already adhering to the sides of the nasal cavity. It is therefore advisable to breathe in an atmosphere, which is full of dust through the nose with closed lips. Yet all danger is not obviated thereby; for we observe especially frequent diseases of these spiratory organs in places, where the air is particularly exposed to many contaminations (cf. § 142).

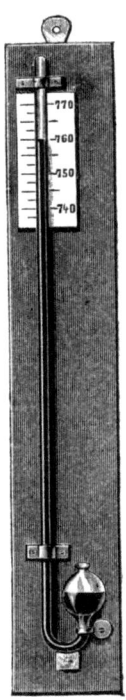

Fig. 15. Barometer.

In towns the air generally is the most contaminated, owing to the large traffic and the great number of factories; the purest air and the healthiest atmosphere is there, where little dust is raised, e. g. in forests and on the seashore.

§ 39. **The climate.** Each place on the surface of the earth stands under the influence of its peculiar meteorological conditions, which are also of importance for the health of man. The sum of these meteorological conditions is called the *climate* of the place. This is judged on the one hand by the average temperature; on the other hand atmospheric pressure, moisture, direction of the wind, rain or other deposits are to be considered. Besides, the frequency of a cloudy sky is of importance, as a clouded sky averts the rays of the sun and somewhat prevents the diffusion of the heat of the earth to the higher layers of the atmosphere.

In general the climate is determined by the geographical position of a place, as the average heat of the atmosphere decreases from the equator to the poles. We distinguish the *tropical* from the *temperate* and *polar climate*. The altitude of a place, through the difference of the atmospheric pressure gives a peculiarity to the *high climate* or the *mountain climate* as peculiar from the *climate* of the *valley*. A relatively small variation of the heat of the atmosphere and a considerable moisture of the air besides frequent rain is a distinguishing characteristic of the sea-coast climate from the *inland* or *continental* climate. Lastly the climate of a place can be essentially different from the neighbouring places, if large forests or mountain ranges afford a protection against the wind, in which the neighbouring place takes no share.

II. Water.

§ 40. **Importance of water.** Water like air is one of the indispensable necessaries of our life. We need it as drinking water, for the preparation of other beverages, in preparing many articles of food, for cleansing our body, our utensils, our dwellings and public places and for many industries. It is an essential part of the tissues of our body; the loss of water experienced by the body through the secretions of the skin, the kidneys, the digestive organs and through the exhaled air requires a regular substitution.

We satisfy our need of water partly by our victuals, which contain water, but for the most part by *beverages*, the consumption of which is caused by the feeling of thirst.

§ 41. Drinking water; its necessary properties. Nature directly offers us drinking water as the cheapest and simplest beverage, but every water is not fit for this purpose. In general we rightly only regard as good for drinking water which is clear, colourless, free from undissolved, swimming matter, which does not possess a strange smell or taste, which is cool and tastes refreshing.

We call water „*hard*" which contains a large proportion of lime or magnesia salt; in opposition to this water is called „*soft*", which is poor in such salts. „Hard" water, which is more pleasant to our taste than „soft" water, is not suitable for washing, because it dissolves badly soap and some dirt-containing substances; also it cannot be used in cooking, as it deposits its salts on the cooking-vessels as so-called „fur", and cannot extract from some food-stuffs the nutriments so well, as „soft" water.

From a hygienic point of view the most important property demanded from drinking-water is that it shall not contain any impurities injurious to health. The above mentioned properties of good drinking-water will generally be some guarantee of its purity; still, water which is unobjectionable as regards appearance, taste or smell may be the carrier of admixtures, injurious to health. Particularly every class of water contains a smaller or greater number of minute living bodies, only visible with a microscope, which are called *micro-organisms*. For the most part these are harmless; still experience has taught that the microbes of contagious diseases can also get into water used for drinking and by means of it can become disseminators of epidemics. In order to obtain a reliable judgment on the fitness for use and innocuity of water, the amount of dissolved matter it contains, as well as the micro-organisms, especially so-called bacteria and the species of the latter must be determined by experts.

§ 42. The source of water. Rainwater. Cisterns. Generally by a knowledge of the *source of the water* we gain already some points for judging of its fitness for use. We distinguish between rain-, spring-, subterranean- and surface water.

44   B. The necessaries of life for the individual man.

Deposited water or meteoric water (cf. § 36) reaches the ground mostly as rain, is poor in saline matter and in conseqence very „soft". As the deposits cleanse the air, — so to say — the first water, falling in a shower or snowfall contains frequently impurities of different kinds, which according to their qualities putrefy under the influence of microorganisms; later falling water it purer. Through rain-water on account of its „softness" is not very palatable, and may even cause digestive disorders, if taken in large quantity; still those who live in waterless regions are compelled to collect it in vessels or in walled cavities, *(cisterns)* and to use it as drinking-water; such cisterns however are easily exposed to contaminations from the surface of the earth.

§ 43. **Subterranean water and springs.** If the rainwater falls on pervious soil, like gravel or sand, it trickles into it and leaves behind in the upper layers of the soil, as in a filter the undissolved impurities, brought with it from the air or the earth's surface. Here the water at the same time takes up certain soluble constituents of the soil as well as carbonic acid from the subterranean air, which is in the pores of the ground. The water, now containing free carbonic acid is able to dissolve partly more earth-minerals, consisting of chalk and magnesian compounds and gradually acquires a „hardness", corresponding to the quantity of mineral matter received. As soon as in the course of its infiltration the water arrives at an impervious soil, (rock, clay or loam) it spreads according to the slope of the soil as *subterranean water*. If the impervious layer is of an undulating form it collects in its deepest places as a subterranean pool or lake; if it has trickled through on the surface of a hill or montain, it can, by flowing down the impermeable layer, reach the bottom of the montain and there appear on the surface as a spring. If the water in its course flows into a space,

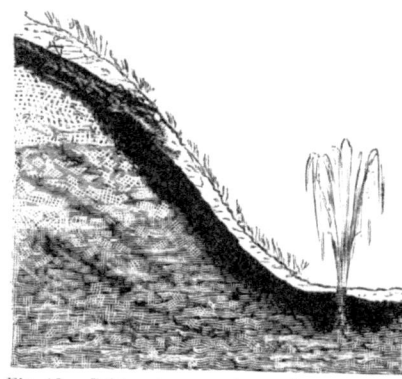

Fig. 16. Subterranean water under pressure spouts in a jet through the aperture, bored in an impervious layer.

bounded above and below by an impervious layer, we see it often spout forth from the orifice with great force, sometimes in a large jet, if the upper layer is pierced from the surface of the earth. (Fig. 16.)

Owing to the filtering nature of the soil subterranean water as a rule is free from bacteria. It contains carbonic acid and mineral substances, has a refreshing taste and on account of its purity is well suited as drinking water. Exception must be made of the water of the so-called ‚*Rasenquellen*' (turf springs) i. e. of such springs, where the water collects so closely under the surface of the earth, that it is neither reliably filtered by the earth, nor sufficiently impregneted with carbonic acid and minerals, nor far enough removed from the influence of solar and atmospheric heat. The water of the *subterranean wells* coming from a moderate depth rises slightly in temperature during the heat of the summer, but is as a rule fit for use; the water of the *mineral springs*, coming from a great depth remains uniformly cool, possesses a pleasant refreshing flavour and is free from bacteria. The last mentioned water can only acquire unhealthy qualities by being contaminated at the spot, where it appears as a spring, or where it is made accessible for use by the buildings near the wells.

§ 44. **Spring-water pipes. Well-Machinery.** Contamination of spring-water may occur, if the water is first conducted into collecting basins or well-chambers in order to be drawn out of these for use or to be conducted by means of pipes to human settlements. In order to prevent pollutions of their contents the collecting basins should be placed as far as possible away from human habitations, and to ward off lateral influxes impervions walls with edges, overhanging the surface of the earth as well as a thick movable cover should be provided. Waterpipes ought to have impervious sides and absolutely tight joiuts.

We distinguish flat- or *surface wells* from *deep wells* (Fig. 17). The water of the surface wells flows from the subterranean water of the uppermost layers of the earth, and hence easily contains injurious ingredients in populous places, the subsoil of which is polluted by the refuse of human habitations. The water of *deep wells* in usually, free from bacteria and decomposed elements of organic matter; but its utility as drinking water, especially in North Germany is more frequently injured than the water from surface wells by a mixture of iron salts, which imparts to the water an inky taste and in the open air causes a gradual deposition of a brownish slime. Various devices have been invented for freeing the deep water from these iron salts.

Owing to the unsuitable construction of a well its water frequently is of a bad quality; particularly the so-called bucket- and pump wells prove objectionable. These are built, by excavating the earth down to the *water bearing* strater and by supporting the sides of the excavated hole by means of beams of timber or masonry. In the hollow or shaft, thus constructed the deep water collects on the floor or ‚bottom' and is raised by means of *buckets (draw-wells)* or *pumping machines (pump-wells)*. If the sides are not quite tight, or if the well is not properly covered — sometimes there is no covering at all — these wells are in a high degree exposed to pollution from the surface or the lateral layers of earth. This happens particularly, if these shaft wells, as is frequently the case in country districts are placed in the neighborhood of dung heaps or cesspools (which are not quite tight) so that the contents of the latter find their way to the water in the well. (Fig. 18.)

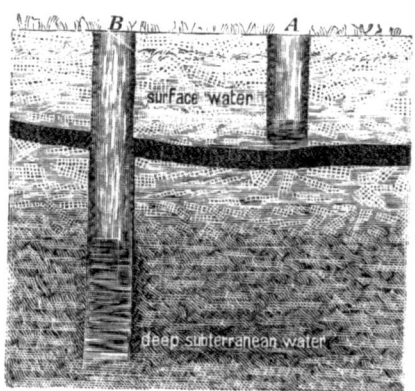

Fig. 17. *Surface and deep wells.*

Even very tight walls of the well give no reliable security for a continued purity, as the substance, used for making tight the walls soon gets cracked and these cracks are usually discovered when the pollution of the water in the well has been already accomplished.

Greater security is afforded by *Pipe wells* (Fig. 19) Abessynian or artesian wells; they consist of an iron tube, which is driven into the earth down as far as the strata, containing the deep water, and is provided with a pumping arrangement at its upper end. The impenetrability of the metal sides excludes every lateral influx into the water.

§ 45. Surface Water. In some places the opening up of the deep water is impossible, or very difficult; either because its basin lies too deep under the surface of the earth, or because the subsoil consists of rock, and cannot be bored without great difficulty and expense; or because the ground-

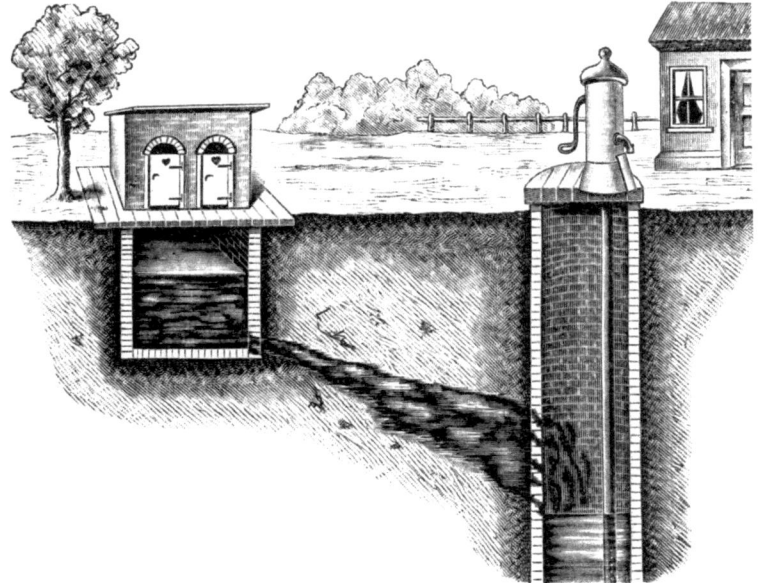

Fig. 18. Pollution of a draw-well by the contents of a neighbouring cess-pool.

water is unfit for use owing to the salts it holds in solution. If in such places springs are not available, the inhabitants are compelled to use *surface water*. By this term is meant the water of *streams*, *rivers*, *lakes*, *ponds* and generally all such water, the level of which is on the surface of the earth. Its value as drinking water is much inferior than springwater or groundwater; it also does not possess in summer the refreshing coolness, as it is exposed direct to the influence of the atmosphere and to the rays of the sun; it is also poor in carbonic acid and mineral substances and generally contains impurities. To the latter belong the excreta and *débris* of aquatic animals and plants, but particularly the refuse of the organic world, living on the borders of the water.

Frequently among the domestic refuse the excreta of sick persons containing the germs of infections diseases are carried to the water. In certain circumstances manifold diseases, epidemics of typhoid and cholera can be caused by the use of surface water for instance: the devastating cholera epidemic which visited Hamburg in 1892 was traced to the unfiltered drinking water of the town, taken from the Elbe.

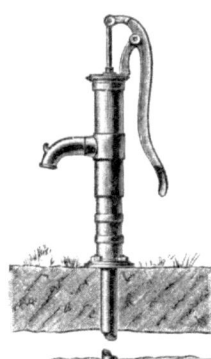

In many stagnant, or sluggishly slow flowing bodies of water such as ponds, ditches, canals or small rivers the resulting pollution shows itself frequently already in the muddy colour, the foul smell and taste of the water; investigations show, that in water in this state there may be found microorganisms up to 100 000 and more per cubic centimetre. The influence of the contamination is diminished, the greater the surface of the water is and the quicker the water is carried away by the current. At some distance from such contamination the water is usually found pure again, it is assumed, that it is able to rid itself of its impurities by means of the so-called *self-purification*. This process takes place on the one hand through the deposition of the filtry matter on the bottom and on the banks of the river, on the other hand by the decomposition of the foreign ingredients, certain noxious species of

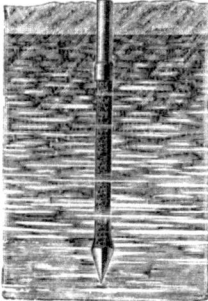

Fig. 19. *Pipe wells.*

bacteria are able however, under certain conditions, which are not yet sufficiently explained to exist a long time in water and transport with it diseases from place to place. Particularly the spread of cholera observed in many epidemics of that disease along the water course of rivers has been connected with a transportation of the cholera germ through the water.

§ 46. Artificial purification of the surface water. Filters.

According to ihe foregoing observations the use of surfac water for drinking or domestic purposes must be considered hazardous; but by certain processes one succeeds to remove more or less the noxious qualities of such water.

The surest way of destroying the germs of disease in water is by *thorough boiling* it, but the water then loses its carbonic acid and with the latter its refreshing taste. Most

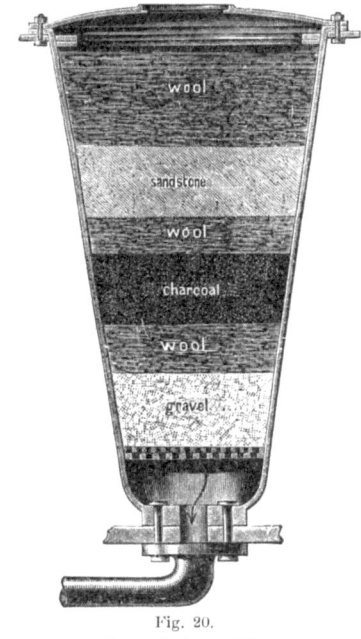

Fig. 20.
Composite house filter.

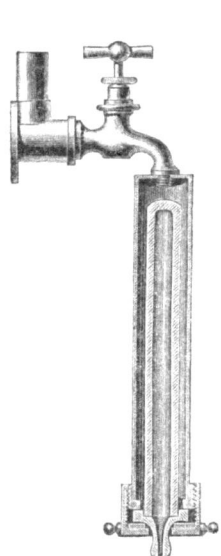

Fig. 21.
Filter silicious marl according to Berkefeld.

chemical means used for purifying water are less successful in killing the germs of disease; moreover the water also loses thereby its taste.

Those processes, based upon the fact, that one allows the water to deposit its impurities by being kept standing for a longer period of time in *clarifying vessels*, only remove the coarser impurities, and therefore are insufficient. Filters however are of greater value. Small filters, so-called house filters (Fig. 20), in the construction of which charcoal, asbestos, porous stones, burnt clay, porcelain or silicious marl (Fig. 21) are employed, can clarify the water very well, but they cannot reliably free it, and then at most only temporarily from the germs, which it contains. For as a growth of microbes takes place in the sides of the filter, the germs, contained in the filtered water increase in a short time, and may be finally more numerous, than before filtration.

More successful are the *sand filters* (Fig. 22), which are used in many towns for purifying water. These sand-filter

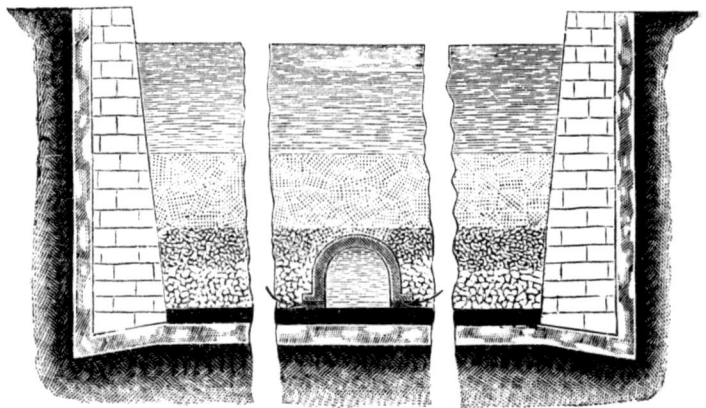

Fig. 22. Plan of a large sandfilter for purifying surface-water.

beds extend over large surfaces, on which are laid in layers, first on the bottous flat stones, then smaller stones, then gravel, lastly fine sand on top. The water, to be purified, filters through all these layers from the top downwards, passes then through canals into pure water reservoirs and from these into the pipes and the water tanks. As the real filtering part of the bed must first be deposited in the form of a fine mud-coating on the surface, the first water, coming from a newly-erected or cleaned filter-bed is allowed to run off waste. When properly built and conscientiously worked the sand-filters retain the coarser impurities of the water completely, and also the bacteria to a great extent; but when improperly constructed or with want of care in their use the results of filtration may be completely lost. Hence in the German

Empire strict government supervision is required in the construction and use of sand filters which are built for the purification of surface water. Many experts however desire, that, whenever possible, deep underground or deep well-water should be exclusively used for drinking water arrangements, and surface-water should be entirely disregarded.

§ 47. **Sea-water.** The kind of surface-water, most widely spread over the earth is the water of the oceans, the sea-water. This is unfit for drinking on account of the high percentage of salt, it contains. If however it is necessary to use it as drinking water, it must be *distilled* i. e. boiled, and the ascending steam conducted through a cool tube. By this process the steam is again condensed into water and the salts remain behind in the kettle. Such water however is only drunk in case of necessity and with some admixtures, as without such additions the water, owing to its want of gaseous and mineral ingredients has an insipid taste and cannot be well digested.

§ 48. **Mineral water.** On its way through the soil (§ 43) water has sometimes an opportunity to take up certain mineral ingredients, especially salt and gaseous substances in large quantities; these ingredients give to the water salubrious qualities. Such water is called *mineral water*. Many kinds of mineral water, which are refreshing beverages are highly esteemed by many healthy and sick persons; these (such as selters-water, containing a large quantity of carbonic acid) are artificially imitated to a large extent by forcing carbonic acid into ordinary water under strong pressure. These imitations may be injurious to health, if bad water is employed in their preparation.

§ 49. **Use of water in removing dirt.** The importance of water for our health is not exhausted by its use as drinking water; on the contrary; of the water, consumed by us, which on the average varies from 50 to 150 litres per day for each individual according to the mode of his life, only three to four litres is used for domestic purposes, inclusive of the portion, indispensably necessary for the preparation of food. The remainder is meant for purposes of cleanliness and for the removal of dirt.

All *elements of dirt*, which are found in our surroundings or adhere to our body, our linen, our clothing can become injurious to our health. As together with earthy matter, they always contain the refuse of the organic world i. e. remains of animals and plants, they usually pass very easily into a state of decomposition and become offensive to us by their smell. Besides, they also sometimes contain the pulverized elements of dried-up expectoration and other excreta of sick persons, which may include germs of disease. Such dirt easily contaminates our food, or when whirled about as dust penetrates through our digestive or respiratory organs into the body (cf. § 182). The surface of our body also affords to these elements of dirt a field for their injurious effects, for they penetrate through the pores into the small glands or through small wounds pass under the skin, mingle with the secretions of the skin-glands and thus find their way into the interior of the body. In this way is explained the origin of many *diseases of the skin*, which appear sometimes as eruptions or small superficial sores, sometimes however, when specially dangerous germs adhere to the dirt-elements cause erysipelas, inflammation, or festering of the cell-tissues (cf. § 215—217).

For the removing of dirt water offers us the best means. We sprinkle the streets with it, we cleanse our dwellings and make use of it for the washing of our clothes, numerous domestic utensils and of our body. In these cases it is also not a matter of indifference, what class of water is used. As cleansing not merely consists in a washing away of the dirt, but is assisted also by the capacity of the water for dissolving other substances, the process succeeds best when soft water is used. For cleaning of our body and of our clothes rain water, and failing it, surface water is particularly esteemed. It ought not to be forgotten however, that contaminated surface-water, i. e. water from sources, which receives outflows from house- or public drains, or which has been used for washing clothes of sick persons, may produce sicknesses in persons, who imprudently come in contact with it. In cases, where, through lack of soft water, recourse must be had to hard water, it is advisable to boil it before using it, because thereby a part of the mineral substances, causing the hardness is separated and the capacity of the water for dissolving dirt elements is increased.

§ 50. Auxiliaries of water for cleansing. Cleansing of

the body and the care of skin and hair. The process of cleansing with water is facilitated by the employment of implements of different kinds (brooms, brushes, sponges, mops, scouring gloves etc.); or by additions, such as soda or sand, which loosen the dirt or make it more easily soluble. For removing fatty dirt-elements *soap*, i. e. a combination of fatty acids and alcalies, at present an indispensable necessity among all civilized nations, furnishes the best aid.

The cleanliness of the body promotes health. For babies and sick persons, who soil themselves with their own excretions, it is particularly essential; but in the case of other persons it also removes many dangerous disease elements, keeps away vermin from the body, strengthens the skin (cf. § 6 and § 23) and imparts to it a pleasant appearance.

For cleansing the body the use of water and soap as a rule is sufficient, in washing our hands the employment of a brush is advisable; in washing a tender skin not too cold water, nor too pungent soap ought to be used. The sweet-smelling ingredients, frequently mixed in soap are not injurious, but quite indifferent as regards health.

The regular cleansing of the hair is also important, as it removes the easily decomposable secretions of the skin glands, which are injurious to the growth of the hair, and also the scurf, constantly separating from the upper skin. Dry hair is with advantage kept soft by mild pomade or hair oil and prevented from breaking off or falling out. All other waters, tinctures, essences, powders, cosmetics and desinfectants, recommended, (e. g. tar or thyme soap) should only be used under medical directions, as preparations of this kind offered for sale (sometimes in a very sensational manner) contain sometimes injurious substances, for instance poisonous metallic compounds or colouring stuffs and moreover are not beneficial to every-one. More particularly is this true of mixtures for colouring the skin and hair, which frequently have a very injurious effect owing to an admixture of lead.

§ 51. Baths and water cures. Besides thorough washing, *bath* offer the most thorough means of cleansing the body; they possess the further advantage of acting in a refreshing, strengthening and sometimes healing manner. Cold baths, especially swimming baths in trustworthy rivers or in a lake or in the sea stimulate body and mind and promote strength.

Warm baths must take the place of cold baths in the case of children, invalids and frequently also of old people, and have besides a soothing effect; they also promote perspiration. Baths in cold and warm mineral water are employed for healing purposes. It is very advisable, not to take a cold bath soon after meals nor until one has become cool; also to dry and dress quickly after the bath in order to avoid chills. The use of impure water for bathing purposes is similarly injurious as its use for drinking.

The healing effects of water are not limited to baths. In the form of *poultices, shower-baths* and *douches* it can also have a beneficial effect and thereby contribute to the restoration of health.

III. Food.

§ 52. Necessity of food. Food supplies the body with the materials which it requires for its growth and for replacing the tissues, used up by the cellular activity. We are induced to take food by the necessity for food, which we call the feeling of being hungry — *hunger*. — The *need of food* is in proportion to the purpose which the food has to fulfil, different in quantity and in quality. As a rule it is increased by an increase in the consumption of materials in the body. Hence during vigorous muscular activity man requires a more considerable supply of food than during repose, and in winter we involuntarily increase our food, because the cold of the surrounding air compels our body to develop more heat; and this must be done by an increased supply of materials to the cells of the body (cf. § 181).

Growing youths or girls on account of the requisite new formation of bodily tissue require a somewhat differently composite kind of food, than is necessary for the sustenance of the grown man. For strengthening the body during reconvalescence after exhausting illnesses, those classes of nourishment, which can be most easily acted on by the digestive organs are most suitable.

§ 53. Composition of food. In accordance with its purpose our food must be composed of all those fundamental primary chemical substances, which have a part in the formation of our body. Among them *nitrogen* is particularly important; for as an essential constituent of the so-called albuminous bodies it assumes an important place in the chemical structure of our body. Next we require *carbon, hydrogen* and *oxygen*. These three primary substances are the chief constituents of a series of non-nitrogenous bodies, which on the one hand supply in great part the material, used up in the cellular functions producing heat, and on the other as fat form also a sort of storehouse of nutriment in the body. This supply affords material for the cellular functions at times when the reception of food in the body is impaired, as by sickness; in this manner it protects the albuminous bodies in the tissues from wearing out and so preserves the organism from a too sudden collapse. *Hydrogen* and *oxygen* moreover in their union as *water* take an important share in the composition of the body, of which 59 per cent in weight consists of water. The other elements which take part in the structure of the body are *chlorine, sulphur, phosphorus, calcium, magnesium* and several other metals, principally iron. The chlorine in its combination with natrium (as salt) forms an important constituent of the blood, while in its combination with nitrogen (as muriatic acid) an active element in the gastric juice. Sulphur is found in all albuminous bodies; phosphorus and calcium form the principal mass of the bones; iron is contained in the red corpuscles of the blood.

§ 54. **Food and nutritive substances.** The above mentioned elements are not received in their pure state into the body in the act of taking food; on the contrary, the *food* which we consume is composed of a series of *nutritive substances* and the latter are formed of the above elements. Besides water and some salts nutritive substances are divided, according to their chemical constitution into a nitrogenous group, the albuminous bodies, and two non-nitrogenous groups, the *carbo-hydrates* and the *fats* (cf. § 21).

The *albuminous bodies* have received their name from the *white of the egg of a chicken,* which is the saturated solution of an albuminous body — the albumin — and which is known by its coagulating through heat. Albuminous bodies form the essential nutriment of *meat*, are found as *casein* in milk and are separated from the latter by coagulation, when it turns sour. Of food-stuffs, belonging to the vegetable kingdom pulse *particularly* contains albuminous matter in the form of legumen and the albumin of grain, called *gluten* is an important constituent of bread.

The *carbo-hydrates* are composed of carbon and the two elements of water and are principally contained in the foodstuffs from the vegetable kingdom. We consume them mostly in the form of *starch*, which forms the essential nutriment in *potatoes* and all farinaceous food. Other carbo-hydrates are the various kinds of *sugar* and *cellulose* (cell- or woody fibre). The former is found especially in vegetable food-stuffs (e. g. *grapesugar, fruit-sugar, cane or beet-sugar)* and also in *milk* as *milksugar*. Some tissues of the human and animal body contain substances, resembling sugar. The cellulose represents an important constituent of vegetable cells and imparts its firmness to wood. It is almost insoluble in the human gastric juice and is therefore of no importance for our nourishment.

The fats are contained both in the animal and in the vegetable foodstuffs; to them belongs lard, butter and oil.

We consume *water* not only in its purity (cf. § 41) and as a solvent of different substances in the form of beverages, but also as a constituent of solid food, as it enters into the composition of most foodstuffs in a greater or less degree. Young vegetables and fresh fruit consist of upward of 90 per cent of their weight of water.

The salts, which convey to the body chlorine, phosphorus, a part of the sulphur and metals, necessary for its structure are found in many foodstuffs. We use Chlorate-Natrium — common salt — as a seasoning for most viands.

Among food-stuffs the albuminous bodies are the most important, because they furnish the nitrogen, necessary for the formation of tissue. The non-nitrogenous food-stuffs supply especially the material, consumed in the cells, and moreover, if partaken in excess lead to an increase in the fat of the body

§ 55. **Choice of food.** The qualities of the nutritive substances contained in food are, in general, unimportant, as regards the feeling of satiety arising from them, because the latter depends essentially on the state of fulness of the stomach. The composition of our food is however by no means a matter of indifference to our well-being; if our body is not to suffer injurious effects, we must supply it regularly with special nutritive substances, in definite proportions and sufficient quantities.

In ordinary circumstances, that food, to which we have accustomed ourselves, under the guidance of natural impulse, corresponds best to the demands of the body. When it is necessary to determine the daily food-supply for a large number of men, where the choice of the individual cannot be consulted (e. g. in the furnishing of food [wholesale] for colleges, barracks, prisons etc.) the calculation is based on the quantity of nitrogen and carbon, which the body gives off on an average in the course of a day through the lungs and the skin as well as with the excreta and the urine. A suitable diet must contribute to the body such a quantity of these elements, as will suffice to replace these daily losses.

By careful investigations it has been ascertained that an adult, well-nourished man in our climate loses every day on an average, when working moderately 18.8 g of nitrogen and 281.2 grammes of carbon in the manner indicated. By supplying about 120 grammes of dry albumin the stated quantity of nitrogen and 64 grammes of carbon would be restored to the body. To replace the missing 217 grammes of carbon, about 280 grammes of fat, or 475 grammes of carbo-hydrates would be required.

In calculations of food however it is to be taken into consideration, that the individual nutritive elements are used differently by the body according to their origin. We receive albumin from food-stuffs, derived from the animal kingdom (flesh, eggs, milk) in a much more digestible form, than from food-stuffs produced by the vegetable kingdom; (pulse and flour) hence, if we wish to satisfy our want of nitrogen by vegetable food only we must consume larger quantities of such food. On the other hand our supply of carbon can be just as easily obtained from vegetable food-stuffs as from animal fat. A diet, composed only of vegetable food *(vegetarian diet)* can satisfy the demands of the body for nutritive substances only on the condition, that very large quantities of food are consumed. But a one-sided diet of this kind leads to the result, that the digestive organs, in consequence of the increased quantity of food must increase their exertions at the cost of the physical development of the entire body. It is advisable therefore, that a part of the necessary nitrogen (a third part at least, from experiments made) should be supplied to the body from the animal kingdom.

In the selection of food the money value (the costprice) of the various food-stuffs has to be taken into account; that of animal food is generally highest.

§ 56. Calculation of daily diet. The facts and considerations just mentioned form the general principles, by whose aid the food supply for large communities of men is usually estimated. In individual cases naturally, the age, the sex, the condition of nourishment and the occupation of the person are taken into account. Furthermore, the season of the year and the climate cannot be left out of consideration in laying down a dietary, as for instance in winter and in cold districts large quantities of fat must be given in order that the heat producing material of the body may correspond to the increased diffusion of heat.

The minimum standard for daily diet has been approximately calculated as follows:

Calculation	Albumin	Fat	Carbo-Hydrates
	g	g	g
Infants up to 1½ years of age	20—36	30—45	60—90
Children from 6 to 15 years of age . .	70—80	37—50	250—400
Male adults at moderate labour	118*)	56	500
Female „ „ „ „	92	44	400
Male adults at severe labour	120—145	100	500
Male persons of advanced age	100	68	350
Female „ „ „ „	80	50	260

§ 57. Preparation of food. Spices and other provisions. If the diet, measured as above is to become a really healthy and strengthening nutritious food, care must be taken on one side for a *change of diet*, on the other hand for a proper preparation of the food. A uniform diet easily produces loss of appetite and disgust. Only by cooking many victuals become edible, because our digestive organs can assimilate many classes of food only in a boiled, roasted or baked form, and some viands even by the addition of stimulating spices only.

By cooking vegetable food the contents of the cells are either extracted or changed into a form more accessible to the influence of the digestive gastric juices; in particular the

---

*) Of these 105 to 106 grammes must be supplied in a form easily digestible by the body. (Cf. p. 56.)

starch is transformed into a more easily digestible paste. In meat also the edible parts are opened up by boiling, as the indigestible fibres, containing the bundles of muscles are thereby loosened, partly they are changed into soluble gelatine, while the albumen coagulates. At the same time the parasites, sometimes to be found in meat such as trichinae and germs of diseases, which enter the meat either from the atmosphere or through lack of cleanliness in slaughtering or in the course of preserving or selling are destroyed or rendered harmless by boiling. The latter result is less certainly obtained by roasting; for in this process the high temperature acts especially on the surface, while the inner parts, owing to the bad conductivity of meat remain more or less raw. However, roasting increases the pleasant taste of the meat, as under the influence of the heat of the oven substances pleasant in taste and smell are produced in the superficial layers of the meat owing to chemical action.

The *seasonings* (salt), and *spices* (pepper, ginger, cloves etc.) have a similar importance for our nutrition, as the so-called *refreshments ("Genussmittel")* e. g. tea, coffee, chocolate, alcoholic beverages. Supplied to the body in moderate quantity and with judicious selection, they increase the digestion, being at the same time agreable to the palate; partaken of immoderately they cause disturbances in the digestive organs and in the functions of other organs.

The *time of the day*, at which we partake of food is also important for our nourishment. Custom and habit have introduced three principal meals a day, *breakfast*, *dinner* and *supper*. During hard bodily or mental work it is advisable to take a not too scanty breakfast shortly after getting up, and to take a plentifull dinner at an hour corresponding to the middle of our working day, i. e. from half an hour to two hours after midday. On the other hand we should partake of far less food for supper, than at either of the two other meals, and it ought to be taken at least $1\frac{1}{2}$ hours before bedtime, so that the work of the digestive organs as well as the other organs of the body may be moderated, and rest granted to them. On the other hand is it advisable to rest a short time after each meal, so that the activity of the digestive organs, required for assimilating the food may not be interfered with by other bodily or mental functions.

§ 58. **Manner of taking food. Care of the mouth and the teeth.** The way, in which we partake of food and drink is also of great importance. Too hot viands and drinks attack the mucous membrane of the mouth, throat and œsophagus and produce disorders in the stomach. After partaking of very cold drinks nausea, vomiting, pain in the stomach and serious disorders of the bowels are observed. It is of great importance, that the food should not be hastily swallowed, but it should be adequately prepared for digestion by thorough chewing and mixing with the saliva. Persons, who cannot do this through lack of good teeth suffer from numerous disorders of the digestive organs. Great attention should therefore be paid to the care of the mouth, necessary for the preservation of the teeth. Good, healthy milk-teeth are a condition for a good permanent „mouthful" of teeth.

For want of proper cleaning scraps of food collect easily between the teeth and in hollow teeth, which there decompose, thereby irritating and giving rise to the pains in the teeth and gums and injuring the good quality of the food by the admixture of their decomposed débris. Care of the teeth aims at preserving for the crown of the tooth its protecting enamel and for the neck and root of the tooth its covering of the gums. In the first place care must be taken for the removal of the tartar, which gathers on the teeth between the neck of the tooth and the gum, uncovers the former, and retains morsels of food in its uneven surface. We should regularly and often rinse and gargle with not too cold water. As an addition to the water so used, some drops of tincture of myrrh, eau de Cologne or an alcoholic solution of peppermint-oil may be useful. We should brush the teeth not only in the morning but also in the evening with powder, which will not injure the enamel. For such purposes preparations, having white chalk or carbonate of magnesia as their basis may be recommended. They may also be perfumed and coloured in innocuous colours. One ought to beware of tooth preparations, which injure the enamel and thereby induce diseases of the teeth. For saving the enamel from injury it is advisable not to expose the teeth to a too great change from hot to cold or to „crack" too hard things; the teeth should also be preserved from the action of powerful acids. We should acccustom ourselves to chew equally on both sides of our mouth. Lastly it is advisable to have one's teeth examined — if possible twice a year — by a dentist; have them freed from tartar, and if necessary treated, as may be required.

The Means of Nourishment.

§ 59. Selection of food for a calculation of our diet. The change of diet required for proper nourishment (cf. § 57) is made possible for us owing to the great number of food substances, available to us. Natural instinct guides us as a rule to a suitable selection. We satisfy for instance our want of fat, sugar and starch by eating with meat a fatty sauce, boiled potatoes and fruit; and similarly we try to supplement a diet rich in starch by fat and albumin as we butter our bread and add cheese to the bread and butter. In still more perfect manner the chemistry of food enables us to regulate the composition of our diet in accordance with the requirements of our body, since that science teaches us the quantitative proportions, in which the individual nutritive elements are contained in different articles of diet.

The coloured diagram (Fig. 23 on the next page) shows at a glance the composition of some important sources of nourishment according to the data supplied to us by chemistry. The names of the chosen food are given under one another; on the right of each name there is a horizontal printed (red) band. The red colour indicates the albumin, contained in the viands; the yellow colour the fat; the blue colour the carbohydrates; the brown colour the indigestable cellular matter; the black shading the salts and the last white space the water, which the foods contain. The length of the individual coloured bands, measured according to the number of divisions, which they occupy indicates in percentages the various nutritive parts, contained in the food in question. Thus in the case of middling fat beef the red colour indicating albumin occupies 21 divisions, because beef contains about 21 per cent of albumin. In lean pork the length of the yellow band covers 7 divisions, from 20 to 27 because in this meat 7 per cent of fat is found.

On the basis of the values, given in the coloured table of the amount of nutritive elements contained in each food, the following diet could be drawn up for a day, which in spite of its simplicity and cheapness supplies the nutritive requirements of an adult man in moderate work according to the dietary standard, given in § 56. One should give: 1. For breakfast: milk, coffee, bread and fat (lard) namely: 200 g thin milk, 240 g rye bread and 25 grammes lard (fat stuffs). 2. For dinner: Beef with „mashed" peas, potatoes and bread; to wit: 150 g middle fat beef; 150 g peas; 400 g potatoes; 10 g fat and 100 grammes rye bread. 3. For supper: Milksoup with rice and bread and cheese; namely: 300 g thin milk; 40 g rice; 20 g cheese (without the fat stuff) and 250 grammes rye bread.

For the whole day would be used:

Foods	Weight in grammes	Price in Pfennige (100 to a sh. 100 = 25 cts.)	Amount of		
			Albumin g	Fat g	Carbo-Hydrates g
Rye bread	600	11	36	3	285
Thin milk	500	5	15.5	3.5	24
Potatoes	400	3	8	0.8	82.8
Beef (moderately fat) . .	150	24	31.5	8.3	—
Peas	150	5	34.5	3	78.8
Rice	40	2	2.6	0.4	31.4
Lard	35	6	0.2	34.7	—
Cheese (lean)	20	2	6.8	2.3	0.7
Note:	1895	58	135.1*)	56.0	499.7

Thus for about 58 (German) Pfennige (= about 15 cents) the constituents of a day's diet can be procured; that is 1895 grammes of foodstuffs, containing 135.1 g albumin, 56.0 g fat and 499.7 carbo-hydrates; while the daily minimum diet for a male adult on moderate labour according to the standard in § 56 requires 118 g albumin, 56 g fat and 500 g carbohydrates. In the daily diet, calculated above about two fifth of the necessary albumin is derived from food-stuffs, supplied by the animal kingdom (meat, milk, cheese), but experience showed that it is sufficient, if one third of the albumin reqired is supplied by these more costly foods (cf. § 55). By the addition of sausage and butter which can be inter-

---

*) Of this about 115 g are usud up by the body.

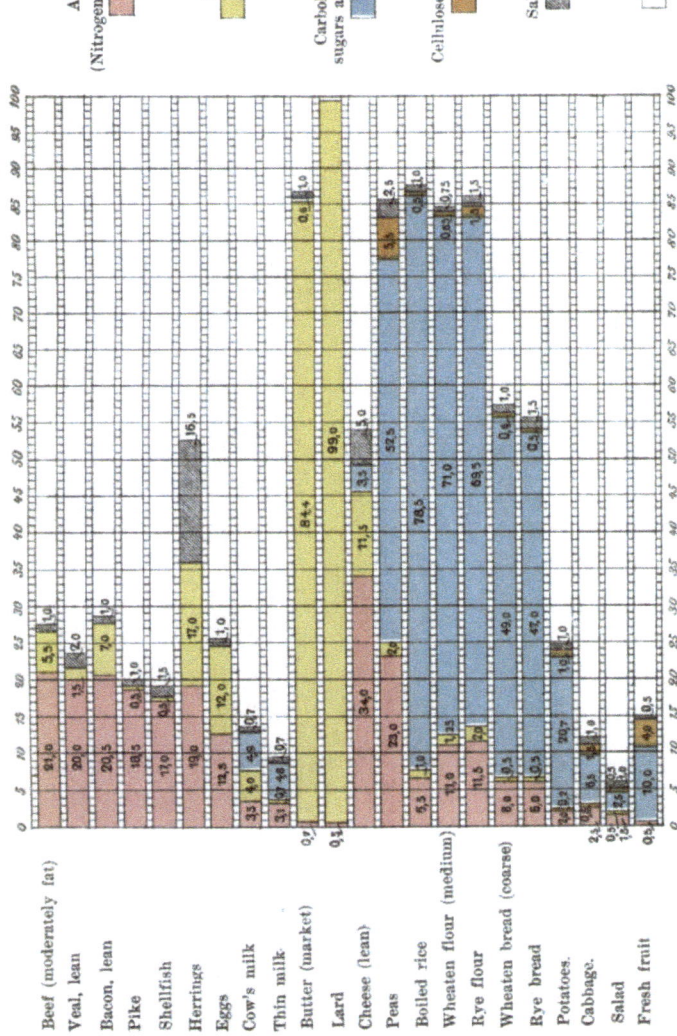

polated with a part of the bread at breakfast and supper this diet can be made still more nutritive, and by adding some „refreshments" e. g. coffee, beer or wine, a greater variety can be obtained.

In deciding on the value of individual food-stuffs it is not sufficient to know their nutritive matter they contain; other properties of the various foods, important from the point of view of health must be taken in consideration. The eating of some vegetables may lead to disorders in the stomach and in the bowels, white bread is more easily digested than black bread, and so on. It is therefore necessary to inquire as to the digestible quality of individual food-stuffs.

§ 60. **Corn and flour.** For the nourishment of larger masses of people the food-stuffs, prepared from corn are of great importance. The plants from which they are obtained, brought by commerce to the most diverse parts of the earth generally flourish best in places, where the climate and the properties of the soil afford favourable conditions for their thriving.

Most kinds of corn belong to the botanical family of grasses and consist like them of root, stalk, leaves and ear. The ear bears the flowers and later on the fruits in the shape of grains of corn. Each grain of corn consists of a shell, formed of indigestible cellular substance and of the kernel, which contains the nutritive substances. By grinding the latter are separated as far as possible from the indigestible cellular material and in the form of *flour* becomes available for further preparation as human food.

The principal nutritive elements in corn are starch and albumin; but sugar, fat and salt are also not absent, so that corn furnishes nutritive elements of every kind. Among the *albuminous* substances *gluten* must be especially mentioned; this makes the baking qualities of flour possible, as it imparts the consistency to dough and thus renders possible the adhesion of the bread while „rising".

Flour is sometimes fraudulently *adulterated* with substances of all kind, of no value at all for nutrition and under certain circumstances even injurious to health. Thus attempts are made to augment its weight by mixing heavy spar and plaster of Paris with it, or to increase its bulk by the addition of the products of overgrown corn, which are less suitable for baking purposes or of the seeds of wild plants. Furthermore the purity of the flour may be injured by want of care in the collection and subsequent treatment of the corn, allowing *foreign seeds* of all kind to mix with it. Adulteration with ergot (a fungus growth, which changes the corn in the ear) is especially to be dreaded, as it produces sometimes serious poisonous effects, when eaten with the flour.

§ **61. Preparation of flour. Pastry.** Flour is used in a great many ways as food. It forms the essential constituent of many *dumplings*, the Suabian „*Spaetzle*", the Bavarian „*Knoedel*", vermicelli and macaroni and is well assimilated by our digestive organs in this form. Many people are fond of *flour-soup* or a kind of porridge for breakfast, but we use *flour* principally in pastry (baked).

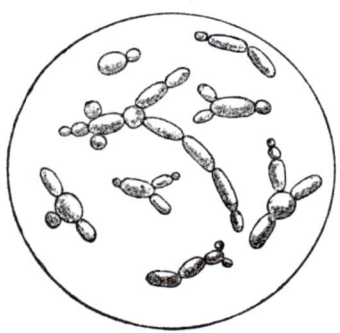

Fig. 24. *Yeast fungi* (greatly magnified).

The process of baking *bread*, the most important product of flour is the following: First of all the flour is kneaded into a dough with water, and this dough is mixed with yeast. Yeast (Fig. 24) is a mass, consisting of minute living vegetable structures, only visible with the microscope, called fungi. The dough commences to „rise"; in its interior numerous bubbles form, it becomes spongy and light; in this condition it is put into the hot baking oven, where it first increases in size, until after a short time the baked bread can be taken out from the oven. In bread we distinguish the hard brown crust from the soft light crumb, pierced by numerous large and small cavities; the colour of the latter, according to the kind of the flour used is sometimes grey and sometimes brown.

The conversion of the dough into bread is brought about chiefly by the agency of the yeast fungi. First of all, these change a part of the starch into sugar, and then immediately give rise to a process of fermentation, by which the sugar is split up into carbonic acid and alcohol. The carbonic acid gas and the alcoholic vapour expand the dough and give it its light spongy character. In the baking oven the yeast fungi continue their fermentative activity, until they die off under the influence of the increasing heat.

Instead of yeast there is sometimes used in the preparation of bread what is called „leaven" i. e. *fermenting dough* from an earlier bread baking. The yeast fungi, in full vital activity in the fermenting dough increase, when fresh dough is kneaded with the latter and thus produce the same phaenomena as pure yeast.

In the fermentation, produced through the agency of yeast or leaven organic acids, especially *lactic acid* are always being formed, which impart a more or less sour (acid) taste to the bread and sometimes produce digestive disorders in the human body after eating bread. To avoid this formation of acids in bread, certain salts are used in the process of baking instead of yeast; these salts possess the property under the influence of heat or by chemical action on one another of producing gases, especially carbonic and accordingly make the dough spongy in similar manner as the yeast. Salts of this kind are contained in baking flour or *baking powders* of different kinds, as supplied by the trade; some kinds of salts e. g. carbonate of ammonia are added to the dough in any case.

§ 62. **Different kinds of bread.** The properties of bread depend on the one hand on the class of grain used, and on the other on the quality of the flour used; in regard to the latter, the manner in which the grain was ground, is important.

It has been found, that the nutritive substances are not equally distributed in the different kinds of grain (corn). Albumin and starch are to be found principally in the outer layers, starch especially in the interior. As in grinding a complete separation of the grain from the husk is impossible, even with the aid of the most perfect milling machinery, a certain quantity of the external layers of grain remain adhering to the cellular husk after milling, forming with it as remnants of mill-stuff known as bran and pollard. Flour is therefore poorer in albumin and salts, than the corn in grain. This is especially the case with the absolutely white flour, which the miller obtains by removing larger quantities of the external glutinous layer of the grain, which impart a gray colour to the flour.

It has been considered, whether it would not be advisable for the purpose of increasing the nutritive value of bread to bake the flour together with the bran, as has been done hitherto in the case of *Pumpernickel;* (black rye bread) and thus turn to account the nutritive substances adhering to the bran. The bran however contains indigestible substances, which not only are a weight for the stomach and the bowels, but also can cause disorders in our digestion by mechanical irritation. While of Munich rye bread 89.9 per cent and of wheaten bread 94.4 per cent of their weight can be digested, only 80.7 per cent of *Pumpernickel* (coarse rye bread) are available for nutriment, a fact, which entirely outweighs the advantage of its greater percentage of nourishing elements. However *Pumpernickel* forms a favourite article of food for many, whose digestive organs are healthy and strong, and nothing can be said against its use, as long as it is well received by the stomach and does not cause disorders in the digestive organs.

Among different kinds of bread we distinguish leaven bread from unleavened, which is baked without the use of yeast or leaven. *Wheaten bread* is the best, and in its preparation some milk or butter is usually mixed with the dough, kneaded from wheaten flour and yeast or leaven. The *black bread*, in some places called *gray bread*, is baked either from rye flour, with the aid of leaven. The dough of *"Kommisbrot"* i. e. the soldier's bread and of the westphalian *Pumpernickel* is prepared from coarsely ground rye leavened, partly mixed with bran. Among unleavened bread we know among other kinds *Graham* bread, which is prepared from coarsely ground wheat, or rye, or maize without the help of anything to make it rise, and *ship's biscuit*, prepared flour without any bran.

§ 63. **Cakes and tarts.** *Cakes* and *tarts* are made in a similar way as bread by baking, but in addition to flour, milk, butter, eggs, raisins, nuts, almonds and spices are mixed with the dough; the raising is effected by yeast, or baking-powder or carbonate of ammonia. The nutritive value and the "digestibility" of these cakes varies very much. As a rule the less coherent and the fatty puff dough is considered particularly hard to digest.

§ 64. **The different kinds of Grain.** As the value of all baker's wares generally, and of bread in particular depends in a great part on the kind of grain, used in their production, it is of no small importance for the sustenance of the people of a country the grain, which grows best in the soil and climate of the country, and therefore can be most cheaply obtained from the agriculturist.

The chief grain of the temperate zone is *wheat.* Its cultivation extends in Europe over Germany, England, Central- and the South of France, Hungary, the Balcan countries, and South Russia. It also thrives in Central Asia, a part of North- and South America, and at the Cape of Good Hope. Most widely spread in our country is the *true* or *naked wheat*, whose grains in threshing fall out "clear" from the ears. In South Germany, especially in Wurtemberg spelt is frequently grown. It can endure a rougher climate and thrives in a lighter soil. It possesses the peculiarity, that its chaff cannot be separated from its grain by the usual method of threshing; but a special milling operation is required for that. Of the other grains *rye*, which stands somewhat lower than wheat in its percentage of albumin is chiefly used in Germany for human food. It endures a colder climate than wheat and a lighter soil and is cultivated in a great part of the temperate zone of Europe, Asia and America.

Wheaten bread is preferred generally in France, England and in the South of Europe and in Germany by the wealthier part of the population. Owing to its lightness, which facilitates its assimilation through the digestive organs, it has in fact some advantages over rye bread, but the latter is an excellent food justly in favour among the largest portion of the population of Germany and the north of Europe.

Another kind of grain, *barley* is largely used for making bread in Northern Russia, Great Britain and Scandinavia. In Germany it is mostly used in breweries; only sometimes it is added to rye- or wheaten-dough to make the bread cheaper. In a prepared form as *pearl barley* we use it for gruel and in soup.

Oats so much esteemed in Scandinavia and in Scotland for making bread is used in Germany as human food only in the form of gruel and groats.

In China, Japan, and Southern Asia generally and in most African countries *rice* in the most widely-spread cereal, and the almost exclusive food of the poorer class of the population. It seems especially fitted for nutrition, because it is cheap, surpasses in nutritive value other equally cheap food, such as potatoes and is completely assimilated by the digestive organs. It has however been observed among the inhabitants of these countries, that an exclusive rice diet has the same disadvantages for the human body as every other exclusive vegetable diet. If a person living only on rice does not consume a relatively large quantity of that food, which again may be unsupportable by his digestive organs, he cannot satisfy his need of albumin; he loses working and vital power and suffers injury to his health much more easily than with a mixed diet.

Maize (kukuruz, turkish wheat) which is distinguished from other grain-corn by the large proportion of fat which it contains, is especially cultivated in southern Europe, Central America and a part of North America. In Italy a part of the population lives almost exclusively on a pastry, called *polenta*, made from maize-flour. In Germany maize thrives but poorly; it is therefore of little importance as human food, just like *millet*, which serves as food for the inhabitants of Egypt and Algiers and East India. In connection with the bread-stuffs *buck-wheat* must be mentioned, though it does not belong botanically to the cereals, but to the family of Polygonacea. In its nutritive value it can be compared to the breadstuffs. Buckwheat (also called *Heidekorn*) has also the advantage of thriving in countries, which on account of cold climate and short summer or the bad qualities of the soil do not allow the cereals to come to maturity. It grows on the cold Sibirian steppes, on the great marshlands of Northwest Germany, and in Poland; it is also well-known in Styria and in North America. Beside its use as bread it is employed as flour or groats for several pastries.

§ 65. **Pulses.** Beside corn, pulses (Leguminous plants) especially *peas*, *beans* and *lentils* form a valuable food, belonging to the vegetable kingdom, as they possess the advantage of being cheap and nutritious. The above mentioned pulse, which we obtain from some plants, belonging to the papilionaceous order contains in their *dried* condition all the nutritive elements in such relatively considerable quantities, that they can in a certain measure replace the food, derived from the animal kingdom. Dried peas, beans or lentils contain about 25 per cent of their weight in albumin and perhaps 50 per cent of starch flour, while green peas and green beans in respect of nutritive value must be reckoned among the green vegetables with regard to their nutritive value, though of a very high value among those. As the *albumin* of pulse, called *legumin* is of a different kind to the gluten of the cereals, and is not adapted to baking, we eat peas, beans and lentils mostly in form of broth or soup. One disadvantage in them are their husks, which consist of indigestible tissue and easily become injurious to the stomach and bowels. It is usual therefore to pass the boiled broth through a sieve, which retains the husks or to use the flour of these pulse, freed from the husk, which can be obtained by the tradespeople. A further disadvantage of pulses is that they cannot be boiled soft in hard or chalky water, because the legumen enters into an insoluble combination with the chalk. In their cooking therefore soft or rainwater must be used, or where these are not to be obtained, the hard water is made soft by the addition of some soda.

The value of pulses as nutritive food is lessened by their absorbing a considerable quantity of water in boiling and thus they occupy a space disproportionate to the amount of nutritive elements, which they contain. Dishes prepared of them, are therefore „heavy" in the stomach and in the bowels. Moreover the repugnance felt by some people against a too frequent meal of peas, beans or lentils is the cause that pulses are in less consideration as food than cereals.

The pulses form the principal constituents of some foods, which are now more or less an ordinary article in trade. To these belongs the "*Pea-sausage*" which was first prepared during the Franco-German war, then the *Hartenstein Leguminose*, prepared from fine flour of rye and lentils and the chinese vegetable cheese *Toa-foo* prepared from grounded peas.

§ 66. **Oil products.** While the nutritive value of the cereals and pulses depends especially on the albumin and carbo-hydrates, they contain other products of the vegetable kingdom distinguished by their fat. Thus from the seeds of some *oil fruits* the fatty oil is pressed, which we are accustomed to add to our dishes. The oil, mostly used for this purpose is olive-oil, which is obtained in southern Europe from the olive, the fruit of the olive-tree. For the poorer inhabitants of Southern France, Italy and Greece it takes the place of butter, while with us it is particularly esteemed in the higher „*cuisine*" in the preparation of salads. In addition *poppy-oil, linseed-oil, sesam-oil* and some other kinds of oil are used, which also grow in Germany. Olive-oil is largely adulterated by American cotton-seed oil. As a substitute for butter the oil produced from the cocoa nut palm has been lately recommended, and they tried to introduce it into our daily use (so-called cokos-butter).

§ 67. **Potatoes. Fresh vegetables.** Besides the products, mentioned already, the vegetable kingdom affords a rich and varied assortment of foodstuffs in various kinds of roots, bulbs, leaves and flowers. The *potato* is known to everybody as a wide-spread food. They grow underground as bulbous thickenings of the potatoe plant, which was brought to our continent by Drake from America towards the end of the sixteenth century. Since about 150 years the potato has been cultivated widely in Germany. The value of potatos depends on their savouriness and their starch; the latter forms about $\frac{1}{5}$ of their weight; but they are inferior to cereals and pulse, as they contain albumin and fat only in small quantities and three fourths of their weight is water. The potato is eminently suited to be an adjunct to other food, rich in albumin and fat, but is not sufficient as an exclusive diet. We digest potatoes most easily in the form of mashed potatoes with milk and butter.

§ 68. **The fresh or green vegetables** have been made perfect from their former state of wild plants through the agriculturist or through the skill of the gardener. To this class belong the green, i. e. unripe or half-ripe fruit of *peas* or *beans*, then among bulbous plants *carrots*, *turnips*, *rape*, *betroot* and *Schwarzwurzel*; all the different kinds of cabbage; *curly cabbage*, *white cabbage*, *red cabbage*, *green or brown kale*, *cowliflower* and *turnip-greens*, finally *spinach*, *aparagus* and *artichokes*. Next to them are the salad plants, *lettuce*, "*Romain*" *endive* and *watercress*, *cucumbers*, *celery*, *onions*, *radishes* and a great number of other plants, (herbs) such as *parsley*, *leek*, *dill* and *chervil*, which are used in the preparation of other dishes, as seasonings for broths and solid food.

All these products of the vegetable kingdom possess only a limited nutritive value, in conseqence of the large amount of water, compared to their other nutritive elements. As is shown by figure 23, cabbage consists $\frac{88}{100}$, salad $\frac{94}{100}$ of their weight and cucumbers even $\frac{96}{100}$ of their weight of water. Nevertheless their importance as food must not be undervalued. We choose them on account of their savouriness, partly of their pleasant odour, not only as an adjunct to other more nourishing food, but because they stimulate the appetite and aid digestion. By means of certain elements, which they contain, especially malic-, wine- and oxalic salts they produce an increased secretion of gastric juices and a vigorous action of the stomach and the bowels. They are by no means quite devoid of nutritive elements; cabbage contain $6\frac{1}{2}$ per cent of carbo-hydrates; green beans $7\frac{1}{2}$ per cent and young peas even 12 per cent; carrots (beetroot) give us a noticeable quantity of ready-made sugar and with green beans and fresh peas we consume albumin amounting to $6\frac{1}{2}$ per cent, resp. $5\frac{1}{2}$ per cent of their weight. Of course, in the usual way of cooking these vegetables, a large part of their nutritive qualities is lost, as the water, in which they are boiled and which contains the soluble effective constituents of this class of food is generally poured away.

As fresh vegetables cannot be obtained at all times and in every place, a method has been invented for preserving them a considerable time in a edible condition and for sending them long distances. For this purpose it is necessary that the vegetables should be freed from the germs of fermentation and decomposition they contain, and afterwards be protected from the ingress of such germs. This end is best attained by exposing the vegetables to boiling-heat in vessels of glass or tin and then at once sealing up the vessels hermetically. By the preparation of dried vegetables and the vegetable tablets, compressed out of these we succeed in lessening the amount of water, contained in the fresh vegetables and chances of their decomposition. Very long time preserved in edible condition, German *Sauerkraut* (a favourite food) can be made by allowing fine-cut cabbage to undersgo thorough fermentation with lactic acid (sour milk).

§ **69. Fungi and Mushrooms.** Food, similar to vegetables are the *edible fungi* or *spores*, which are consumed by the population in many districts of Germany, Bohemia, Hungary the Balcan countries, Upper Italy and Russia.

We know about 40 different kinds of edible fungi. Of the group of the cap-fungi the most valuable edible fungi are the true orange agaricus, the golden agaricus, the yeast fungus, the hawk weed, the yellow agaricus, the *mushroom* and the yellow *Boletus*. Among the sack-fungi the most valuable are the *truffles* and *morels;* among the puffballs the red and yellow puff balls and the common *Bovist*. The two last named fungi are suitable for cooking only in their earliest development, because they fall into powder, when getting old. They are sometimes fraudulently offered as truffles as well as the injurious potato- or hart-bovist.

Among the poisonous fungi, which could be mistaken for the edible are the *Agaricus piperatus* puff-ball, the *toad-stool* and the poisonous orange agaricus, belonging to the cap-fungi and the turban top of the sack species, which often cause poisonous results owing to their resemblance to morels. The folded morel, which is sometimes present as an adulteration of the true morel is, when fresh, poisonous, but may be rendered harmless by boiling with water. It should therefore, after boiling be washed and eaten withous its sauce.

Some of the fungi, as for instance morels and yellow agaricus grow chiefly in forests, others, as mushrooms principally in meadows and grassy places. Fungi are collected either in the spring, like the morels, or in the latter part of summer and in autumn like the mushrooms; they appear in large quantities more particularly after warm rain. In collecting them they should not be torn out by their roots, but cut off at their lower part and the stalk covered with earth, so that the part remaining behind in the ground is preserved for further growth. Fungi, which have been nibbled at by insects should be avoided, and young ones should be collected. As fungi quickly decay and thus become injurious to health, it is advisable to cook or dry or preserve them soon after they have been collected. This is especially so with fungi that have been collected during rain, because these quickly decompose under the influence of the rain water which they have absorbed.

Most fungi have a composition similar to that of fresh vegetables; as however they contain particularly large quantities of nitrogen and are completely free from starch, it has been assumed, that they could afford a substitute for animal food, especially for meat. This is however an error; fungi are not easily digested, because they contain their nitrogen only partly in the form of albumin, partly in the shape of other compounds, that cannot be employed in nutrition and therefore are only incompletely assimilated in the human bowels. It is therefore correct to consider fungi similar to vegetables in respect to their value as food.

The non edible fungi owe their injurious effects to *strong poisons*, among which the *Muscarin*, the poison of the toad stool has been carefully examined. The ignorance in distinguishing between edible and poisonous fungi has already resulted in many cases of illness and death, and therefore the sale of fungi has in some countries been placed under police supervision. In Austria there are specially appointed "market-helpers" for this purpose. The marks between edible and poisonous fungi habe been repeatedly made known publicly, because the popular tests are uncertain and deceitfal. For neither in the presence of milky juice nor in the bright colours, nor the glutinous touch of the cap, just as little as in the turning black of an onion, boiled with them, nor in the fact that salt becomes yellow, nor that a silver spoon dipped into the juice turns black, is there a sufficient and reliable indication for deciding on the properties of fungi. We can be quite certain only, if we acquire a thorough knowledge of the distinctive marks of the edible and poisonous fungi and reject all doubtful fungi.

The injurious effect of eating poisonous fungi reveals itself generally after one to four hours. Pains in the limbs, stomach and bowels are followed by vomiting together with nausea and cramp; pain increases, violent thirst, palpitation of the heart, dizziness and faintness set in; finally death results from cessation of the heart's action, stupefaction and convulsions. In the case of some fungi, as for instance puffball fungus the poison begins to act only after eight to forty hours which decreases the hope of help beeing possible owing to the spread of general poisoning. The treatment in cases of poisoning by fungi is similar to that given in § 236 for poisoning by so-called narcotic poisons. The stomach should be directly emptied by exciting vomiting, and medical advice should be at once called in.

§ 70. **Fruit.** *Fruit* occupies an intermediate position between nutritive food and refreshments. We eat *fruit* less for the purpose of food than of refreshing ourselves, while at the same time the usually pleasant odour delights us. However fruit contains also nutritive food, especially sugar and also substances, which help digesting. To the latter belong the vegetable acids, which cause the flavour of fruit.

We distinguish three groups of fruit: 1st *Kernel-fruit*, like apples, pears, quinces and oranges. 2^{d} *Stone-fruit,* as cherries, plums, apricots and peaches. 3^{d} Berries, as grapes, white currants, gooseberries, strawberries, raspberries, huckleberries and cranberries. To these groups may be added the *shell-fruit*, distinguished by the carbo-hydrates and fat which it contains, such as *almonds* and *nuts;* then finally a group of different fruit like *melons, figs, pineapples* and bananas. With few exceptions, among which are quinces and cranberries fruit can be eaten fresh as well as cooked. To preserve fruit in edible condition for a longer period of time, various devices are employed as with vegetables. By drying under gentle heat we obtain dried apples, pears and plums and from grapes we obtain raisins; by boiling with sugar and keeping them in airtight vessels we obtain preserved fruit. The *juice,* pressed from *cherries* and *berries* is boiled with sugar to make *fruit-jelly.* Lastly, by thickening the juice of *apples, pears, plums* and grapes so-called fruit *"Kraut"* (in the Rhineland) is made in many districts. All these products retain their vegetable acids and thus act on our digestion in the same manner as fresh fruit; but, as by drying and preserving the amount of nutritive elements, especially of sugar is proportionately increased by the removal of water, they surpass fresh fruit in nutritive value. Lately a less valuable substitute for fruit-

Kraut, consisting of peel and core from American apples has been introduced by the tradesmen.

§ 71. Sugar. We find in the juice of fruit and in many other parts of some plants various kinds of sugar (cane-, grape-, fruit-sugar). In ordinary use we employ the kind of sugar, called *cane* or *beet sugar*. It was originally made from the juice, pressed out of the *sugar-cane*, that grows in the tropics; but at present it is obtained in Germany, France, Belgium and Russia from the *juice of the beet-root*, after the latter has been cut up, soaked in lie and compressed. According to its greater or less purity, beet-root sugar is called refined sugar, melis (loaf) lump sugar or soft sugar. If one allows a solution of beet root sugar to crystallize on threads, suspended in it we obtain "*sugar-candy*".

Grape sugar is also used to sweeten food and refreshments. But for this purpose it is made on a large scale from potato starch by the action of dilute sulphuric acid, and not from the juice of grapes or other fruit. The product, obtained by this process, called *starch-sugar* is brought into trade both in the solid state as well as in a liquid state, the latter known as *starch-syrup*, or capillar-syrup.

Sugar has great importance for the human nutrition; for it is directly absorbed in the body as nutritious food and need not be first separated by the digestive organs to become an element of nutrition.

A minor product obtained in the manufacture of cane sugar is colonial-sugar *(molasses)*, which is used in cooking and which children are fond of eating with bread instead of butter. The so-called "*barley sugar*" is produced as a glassy mass, if freshly made thick sugar-syrop is boiled and then allowed to cool very quickly.

As the manufactured sugar possesses ordinarily a light yellowish colour, some blue ultramarine is frequently added to make it appear white. Sugar, thus coloured is unfit for preserving fruit, as the ultramarine produces with the vegetable acids, contained in fruit foul-smelling and poisonous sulphureted hydrogen gas.

Besides the sap of fruit, sugar-cane and beet root the saps of various other plants (maple etc.) contain sugar. Similarly the animal kingdom affords us a class of sugar, the sugar contained in milk (*milksugar*). For some time artificial sweetening-stuff has been employed for the purpose of sweetening food. Their sweetening power is higher than cane- or beet sugar, but their nutritive value is less. Their use is advisable only in the case of some illnesses. The use of saccharine and other artificial sweet-stuffs in the preparation of food and luxuries is regulated by the Imperial Law dated 6 July 1898 (cf. § 144).

§ 72. Honey. Closely related to sugar is *honey*. It consists chiefly of a mixture of grape sugar and fruit sugar; it contains moreover water as well as small quantities of albumin, formic acid and salts. It is sucked by the working bees from the flowers of many plants and brought to the beehive, from the honey comb, of which it is obtained. The best honey is the virgin honey, which flows spontaneously out of the comb, or is separated from it by the aid of a honey-shaker. The rough honey, obtained by squeezing and heating the honeycomb is of less value. Adulterations of honey with starch-syrop are frequent.

Honey is not only a valuable means of nutriment on account of the sugar which it contains, but also as an aid to digestion. We use it ordinarily in its purity with bread or with rolls; it is also baked with flour and spices into a cake, called spice-cake or gingerbread. By the fermentation of a mixture of honey and water is produced *mead*, a beverage, much favoured in former times. In some rare cases poisonous effects have been observed after eating honey, that was probably collected by the bees from poisonous flowers.

§ 73. Confectionary. Honey, sugar and starch-syrup are used in many ways in the preparation of the bonbons, gingerbread, and other sweetmeats, sold in confectioner's shops. All these *confitures* are popular with many persons on account of their pleasant taste; still a frequent and large consumption of them may lead to diseases in the teeth and disorders in the digestive functions and sometimes these sweetmeats contain unhealty adulterations. Thus some confectioners increase the weight of their cheaper wares by adding entirely indigestible and therefore injurious substances, such as heavy spar plaster of Paris and similar substances. The almond flavour of some confections is produced by means of oil of Mirbane which possesses poisonous qualities.

§ 74. Food from the animal kingdom. Compared with the foods, derived from the vegetable kingdom, already mentioned above, the nutritive foods from the animal kingdom have the advantage of supplying us with albumin and fat in a form especially easily assimilated by our body. Most of these foods are also distinguished by the high percentage of nitrogenous, nutritive elements, which they contain, many also by their richness in fat, while carbo-hydrates are altogether wanting in them. But; there is one food derived from the animal kingdom, which contains all the nutritive qualities necessary for the continued existence of the body, and which therefore is alone able to maintain and promote the growing of the body in the first period of life. This food is *milk*.

§ 75. **Milk.** *Milk* is secreted by the lactic glands, which in animals are called *udders*. We generally use cow's milk, but among other nations, and even among ourselves the milk of the sheep, the goat, the horse and the ass is used for human nutrition.

Cow's milk is a white fluid, which indicates a larger or less percentage of fat by presenting a yellowish or bluish tint; it possesses a sweet taste, and consists of water, solid constituents dissolved in it, and fat. In the solid constituents are included various *albuminous* bodies, among them especially *casein;* then of the *carbo - hydrates milk - sugar* and some salts. The fat floats in the milk in the form of innumerable small globules — called *butter-globules* — which are only visible with a microscope. In the stomach the casein of the milk at first coagulates in fine flakes, which are again dissolved by the gastric juice.

On account of its solid constituents milk is heavier than water, but every milk has not the same weight. The weight of a litre milk varies from 1026 g to 1040 grammes; a litre of water weighs 1000 grammes.

The proportion by weight, in which the various constituents are contained in milk is influenced by the nutritive character of the fodder, supplied to the animals, particularly by the quantity and digestibility of the nitrogenous substances furnished for consumption, by the quantity of water and salt consumed by the animals, by the length of time, elapsed, since the secretion of the milk began, by the frequency and thoroughness of the milking, and from the special qualities of the cow (the breed).

The contents of fresh cow's milk varies as follows:

	Water	Casein	Other albuminous substances.	Fat	Milk-Sugar	Salts	
From	83.87	1.17	0.04	2.04	2.00	0.34	per cent of the total weight.
To	91.50	5.74	5.04	6.17	6.10	0.98	

In general cow's milk contains more casein than human milk, but less sugar and about the same quantity of fat as human milk. Therefore, if it is desired to replace mother's milk by cow's milk for babies, it is advisable to dilute the latter for the purpose of obtaining an equal proportion of albumin, and also to add some sugar (best is milk-sugar). The dilution is the more necessary, as the albumin of cow's milk is less digestible than the albumin of mother's milk, and by its greater quantity demands an increased activity of the gastric juice of the baby, which may lead to severe illness (cf. § 157). General directions as to the quantity of water, to be added cannot be given, as in every special case the age, the state of health, the strength etc. of the child must be taken into consideration.

During the first days of *milk-secretion* the udder of the cow furnishes so-called *unripe, unmatured* or biestmilk, which is distinguished from the mature milk by a greater quantity of albumin, and less sugar. It has the appearance of a thick yellowish fluid which coagulates, when being boiled and is unfit for food.

Even the matured milk may, under certain circumstances possess qualities, by which it is diminished in value, or even becomes injurious to health. When fed on fodder, lacking in nutriment or in consequence of diseases the cows yield *watery milk*, which is poor in albumin and fat and shows a bluish colour. *Blood-coloured* milk may appear after the eating of sharp, resinous fodder, or in certain diseases and after injuries to the udder. If the udder is inflamed, the milk brings with it flakes, matter, or lumpy coagulated substances; if certain bitter plants have been consumed by the cow, the milk has a *bitter taste*. Some *medicines*, which may have been given to the cow, and finally *disease germs*, particularly of cattle murrain, which corresponds to tuberculose in men (cf. § 229) and of the foot-and-mouth disease (cf. § 223) may pass into the milk and become injurious, if used by human beings. Disease germs can also pass into the milk from the hands of the milkers, or generally through lack of cleanliness in the dairy. All such impurities are not easily perceived in the milk; it is therefore advisable to render them innocuous by boiling; all milk, of whose absolute purity we are not reliably informed (by knowing the state of the dairy etc. for instance) ought to be heated to boiling point before being used.

§ 76. Formation of cream and souring of milk. A distinction is made between fresh (fat) cow's milk and skim milk, which has been deprived of its fat for the most part. As the fat in milk, which is left standing undisturbed rises to the surface owing to its lesser weight, there forms gradually, most quickly in warm weather a *layer of cream* on the surface of the milk; this cream contains about 22.46 per cent of its weight in fat; about 4.22 per cent casein, 3.88 per cent of milk-sugar and 0.4 per cent of salts. If this layer is drawn off, or if the milk is skimmed by means of special appliances (centrifugal separators) the skim milk remains behind, which contains but little fat, and is heavier than fat milk and shows a bluish colour.

Besides the formation of cream other changes take place in milk, when left standing for some time. Under the influence of bacteria, which get into the milk, the milk-sugar changes into lactic acid and carbonic acid; at the same time the milk thickenes, as the casein separates itself from it. In this way *sour milk* or *curdled milk* is formed. Some special kinds of microscopic fungi can destroy milk in such a degree, that it becomes quite unfit for use and even injurious to health. Thus are produced those kinds of decomposed milk, called blue, red, mucous and thready milk.

§ 77. **Preserved milk.** In various ways milk can be preserved, its *freshness kept up* for a long time. Milk is *pasteurised* (a process, first used by Pasteur, a celebrated French analytical chemist) by being heated up to 70^0 to 75^0 C. for at least half an hour and then letting get cool again. By this means the germs, causing milk to turn sour, are killed and the milk retains its original taste; but diseasegerms, which may have been in the milk are not destroyed with certainty.

In *sterilisation* (i. e. destroying of germs) the milk is heated up to 100^0 C. for a longer period, or to 120^0 C. a shorter period of time. According to the Soxhlet process the flasks, filled with milk for the purpose of sterilizing infant's milk are heated at least a quarter of an hour. Under the influence of this *sterilisation* the germs of disease, which are in the milk die, but the milk suffers some changes, which diminish its taste. If the milk, thus treated is to be preserved for a longer period of time, it must be kept cool and in hermetically closed vessels. By the process of boiling and afterwards *freezing* it, milk can also be preserved.

Condensed milk is produced by vapourizing the water; in some factories it is preserved for a longer time by the addition of cane-sugar. By mixing condensed milk with flour, specially prepared from grain or pulse *infants food* is prepared, which in some cases is a very good nourishing food for children.

§ 78. Adulterations of milk. It is to be regretted that milk is oft *adulterated*. Particularly its quantity is increased by dilution with water or skim milk, or its value is lessened by removing the cream. Besides, attempts are made to keep it fresh by adding soda, bicarbonate of soda, boracic acids, salicilic acids etc.

§ 79. Butter. Butter is obtained from milk by thorough churning of the slightly-soured or sweet cream, which causes a separation of the fat, it contains from the fluid constituents. The fatty lumps thus produced are collected, washed and kneaded into butter. In many parts of the country they try to attain a greater keeping quality of the butter by adding salt to it. The butter made from sweet cream in distinguished by its agreable flavour from that made from soured cream, but it does not keep as well as the latter. The table butter intended for eating ought to contain as little casein and water as possible; must be hard and conform in its composition to the values given on the coloured diagram. (Fig. 23). As cooking butter less valuable butter may be used without injury. Preserved butter is made by removing all casein from the fresh butter by repeated washings, by mixing with it a larger quantity of kitchen salt (from 3 to 10 per cent) of its weight and then packing it into barrels (firkins). In South Germany and in the adjoining mountain districts it is the custom to remove the casein from the butter by melting; in this way the so-called melted butter (also called "cattle fat", is obtained. The more or less *yellow colour of the butter* depends on the quality of the fodder, but it is sometimes artificially increased. The melting point of butter lies between 31 and 36° C., rarely between 41 and 42° C.

Fresh butter on account of its pleasant flavour and its *digestibility*, in which it excells above all other kinds of fat, is a popular food. Old butter easily becomes *rancid*, volatile fatty acids being formed, which not only destroy the taste of the butter, but also irritate the mucous membranes of the digestive organs and thus cause nausea.

The remnants from milk, after butter has been made, are called *butter-milk;* this contains of nutritive elements especially casein and milk-sugar and possesses a gentle purgative action.

Attempts have been made to replace butter by cheaper productions, known as artificial butter or margarine. In their manufacture the easily melted constituents (oleo-margarine) are removed from heated beef fat by pressure. The stearine, which only melts at a higher temperature remains behind in the fat and is applied to other purposes, especially to manufacturing candles. The oleo-margarine is mixed with various vegetable oils (sesame oil, earth nut oil, cottonseed-oil) and pigs lard and then worked up with milk, to margarine. In the German Empire margarine may only be sold by that name. (cf. § 144.)

§ 80. Cheese. Besides butter, milk yields us an important food, *cheese*. This is made by allowing the casein in the milk to coagulate, separating it from the *whey* left behind and then submitting it to further treatment according to the kind of cheese required. We distinguish between *superfatty cheese*, which is made from fresh thin milk and the cream of the previous evening's milk; *fatty cheese*, in whose preparation ordinary milk is used, and *lean cheese*, in the making of which skim milk is used. Besides there is *pressed* and *unpressed cheese*.

By means of the cheese press the cheese is freed from those particles of *whey*, by whose fermentation it would otherwise decompose and at the same time obtain a sharp unpleasant taste. The mild taste of many kinds of cheese is due especially to repeated and careful working up and pressing out. Unpressed cheese must be eaten fresh, unless it is preferred to let it mature, that is to pass it into a state of fermentation, and then subject it to a further process, by which it becomes durable and acquires a strong taste. Into this chapter belongs the treatment with mouldy fungi (Requefort), sour beer, "*Trebern*", hops (beer-cheese) certain herbs, brandy, wine, oil, butter, moist straw, nut leaves etc.)

Furthermore; many differences between various kinds of cheese depend on the manner in which the coagulation of the casein in the milk is produced. The separation of the casein is effected either by heating the milk, which has already become somewhat sour (*sour milk cheese*) or by the addition of acids etc. most frequently by calf-rennet. According to the kind of milk used, we distinguish between *cow, goat, sheep* etc. cheese; according to its external qualities we call the various kinds of cheese: *streaked, soft, hart or grated cheese*.

Cheese is sometimes artificially coloured; e. g. Edam cheese is usually coloured red outside. Adulterations of cheese are seldom made; still there is *margarine cheese*, which is made from skim milk and several fats not obtained from milk. Old cheese easily decomposes, moths or maggots settling in it.

In consequence of its richness in albumin, cheese possesses double or triple the nutritive value of some kinds of meat; but it is easily digested only, when it has been chewed very well. The sharp taste of many classes of cheese (e. g. Roquefort) confines their use to occasional small quantities; such classes of cheese as Roquefort for instance are eaten chiefly as a savoury after meals. They excite the digestive organs to a larger secretion of their juices in the same manner as spices or condiments and thus facilitate the digestion of foods, eaten before.

The *whey* which remains behind in the preparation of cheese possesses also an effect towards facilitating the digestion and therefore is employed in the so called *whey-cures*.

§ 81. Eggs. Besides milk and its products *eggs* are one of the most important articles of food from the animal kingdom. Hen's eggs are most frequently eaten; duck's eggs, goose eggs, and turkey's eggs are used less frequently, while pheasant's eggs, gull- and plover's eggs can be eaten only as dainties on account of their high price.

The *Hen's egg* consists of the *yolk*, the *yolk skin*, the *white* (Albumin), the *shell skin* and the *shell*. In the *yolk*, immediately under the yolk-skin is a small white disc, the germ-disc (eye of the egg). The white of the egg is a sticky fluid. The shell skin consists of two layers, which separate from one another at the thick end of the egg, and thus enclose a space of air. The shell consists almost entirely of carbonate of lime; it is pierced by fine holes, which allow free passage to the air.

A hen's egg weighs on the average sixty grammes, of which two thirds the white, and one third the yolk weigh. From the albumin it contains it corresponds in nutritive value to about 40 grammes of fat meat or 150 grammes cow's milk. The fat it contains amounts to somewhat more than one-tenth of its weight; it contains however no starch and no sugar.

The albumin of the egg coagulates as soon as it is exposed to the gastric juices. For this reason a hard-boiled egg, in which the albumin has already coagulated is not in itself more difficult of digestion than a raw or a soft-boiled egg. However, the circumstance, that the albumin of the latter coagulates in the stomach in thin flakes which present a greater surface to the action of the digestive juices favours digestion in ordinary circumstances.

Fresh eggs are savoury, clear and transparent; old eggs are dull, non-transparent and, when bad have a bad, foul smell. Fresh eggs are heavier than water and therefore sink in it. Rotten and incubated eggs float on the surface, because they contain air.

In order to keep eggs for a long time, they must be placed in frames provided with holes, in which they are put with the thinner and downwards. But it is necessary that the egg-shell is intact and that the egg was not already incubated. Eggs can also be kept fresh by rubbing them over with lard, oil, molten wax, shellac, varnish or waterglass or by putting them in melted paraffin, ashes or dry sand. All these devices purpose the keeping out of fresh air and moisture.

Eggs sometimes contain foreign bodies, such as feathers, grains of insects, small worms (so-called "intestine worms") coagulated albumin or blood and other substances, which cause them to "go bad" quickly.

§ 82. **Meat.** By meat, as food we understand the edible parts of animals, especially the muscles with the fat. Of other parts and of the intestines the heart, lungs, liver, kidneys, spleen, brain, tongue, sweetbread, breast and blood are also used for food. The animals, whose flesh we particularly use as food are the *ox*, *sheep*, *pig*, *poultry*, *game* and *fishes*.

The eminent importance which meat possesses for human nutrition is due to the relatively large quantity of albumin and the easily digestible form of this albumin; besides; it contains salts under certain circumstances large quantities of fat; but it contains no carbo-hydrate.

The good quality, savouriness and nutritive value of meat depend on the class, age and sex, on the kind of feeding and manner of foddering of the animals, as well as on the body from which the meat is taken. As a rule the meat from young animals is soft, tender and of a pale-reddish colour; that of older animals is generally deficient in fat, tough and darker coloured. This is especially the case with poultry, which is most tender and savoury in the first year of the life of the bird. By a certain method of foddering, called fattening the proportion of water, contained in the meat is decreased, while the fat is increased. The peculiar flavour of game, known as *haut goût* is due to a peculiar chemical quality of the flesh as well as to the beginning decomposition, which sets in rapidly especially in the case of animals, which have been hunted.

The lean meat of the calf, the chicken, the pigeon, which is called *"white meat"* from the colour, it assumes after boiling, as well as game and tender, lean beef are most easily digested, while the other kinds of meat make higher demands on the activity of our digestive organs. Very fat and sinewy meat is the most difficult to digest. The heart, tongue, liver kidneys and brain of our slaughtered animals are generally digested without difficulty, though they cannot be reckoned among the food most easily assimilated. But the luxury of the lungs of cattle and sheep and pâte de foie gras is advisible to such persons only, who rejoice in very healthy organs of digestion.

§ 83. Flesh of diseased animals. Parasites of meat.
From the diseases of animals their flesh suffers various changes. It can be bloody, watery or purulent; it may contain animal or vegetable parasites. Of the first-named the *Trichina* (spiralis), cysts, the case-worm, liver-fluke, lung-worms etc. are the most important.

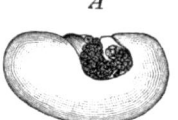

Fig. 26.
Cyst-Germ, with inturned head.

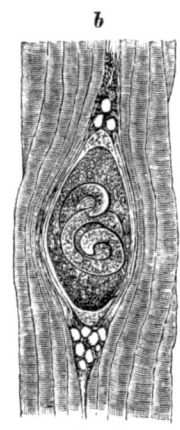

Fig. 25.
Trichina encysted. Greatly magnified.

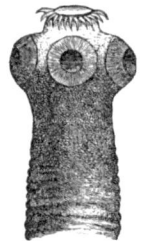

Fig. 27.
Head of swine-cyst.
(Greatly magnified.)

The *trichina* is a small worm, mostly found in swine. In its undeveloped or larva condition it is found in the flesh of the muscles, and there it is enclosed in small capsules (fig. 25) embedded in the muscular fibres. After some time they become like chalky points, and are visible to the naked eye as small white dots only. The trichina remains alive for a long time in its chalky capsule, and withstands long the influence of cold as well, as mild pickling and curing. If meat, permeated by *trichinae* is eaten uncooked by men, the capsules are dissolved by the gastric juices, and the worms thus set free increase to extraordinary large numbers within a very short time in the intestines. The young trichinae pass through the sides of the small intestines into the muscular flesh and roll themselves up there to get into capsules again. By these wanderings and the breeding of young trichinae in the human body cases of diseases are produced, which exhibit themselves as digestive disorders (nausea, vomiting, pains in the bowels, diarrhoea), furthermore pain in the muscles and fever, and not unfrequently death ensues.

Among *cysts* the most important kinds for us are the *pig - cysts* and the *cow - cysts*. They appear as small vesicules (blebs), varying in size from a pea to a bean, and contain water; through the side of the blebs the crushed in head of the animal appears as a yellowish spot of the size of a hempseed. (Fig. 26.)

In this we observe by the microscope four suckers; in the swine-cyst besides there is a double-hooked crown-shaped ring. The cysts in swine and cattle generally appear in the connecting tissues, which divides the single muscle and groups of muscles. (Fig. 27.) If they are eaten with raw meat, they attach themselves firmly by their "suckers" and "hooks" to the inner sides of the bowels, so as to grow into the *tapeworm*, (Fig 28) sometimes several metres long, new members (limbs) being constantly added to the head. The presence of a tape-worm in the intestines can cause many disorders, such as pain in the bowels, nausea, costiness, diarrhoea and produce serious troubles of the digestive organs.

Actinomices causes sometimes swellings in cattle and swine, in which they lie scattered as small yellow dots of about the size of a grain of gravel.

In swine flesh other structures, similar to those actinomices are frequently met with. Even in men actinomices are sometimes the cause of severe illness, united with festering, which attack the lungs, lymphatic intestines and bones. Sometimes the illness is caused by a decayed tooth. A „transfer" of these actinomyces to men by eating the flesh of animals, affected by them does not take place according to our experience up to now.

The germs of some other illnesses, such as anthrax and other diseases of animals can also be found in meat, and besides some poisonous substances, which have been eaten by animals can be conveyed into their flesh.

§ 84. **Decayed meat. Inspection of meat.** Besides the diseases of slaughtered animals, other circumstances, such as decomposition, mouldiness or improper treatment (blowing up)

III. Food.

may injure the relish, the quality of being eaten and the value of meat.

All meat is to be considered as tainted, which is discoloured, unclean, dirty, possesses an offensive smell or otherwise displays unusual qualities. Approaching decomposition is frequently indicated by a dark, purple colour in the meat. If meat is calculated by tainted conditions or changes to cause a disturbance of our health, it has a nauseating character, or it comes from animals, which immediately before slaughtering were suffering from diseases, communicable to men, it must as a rule be rejected as *injurious to health*. To protect the population from using such meat, there is often a rule in some countries, that all meat, before being allowed to be offered for sale, must be examined by special experts *(meat inspectors)* whether it is fit for use as human food. In such an examination the entrails of the animals must be specially examined, as in most cases the disease can be revealed only by the condition of the animals intestines. In Germany by an Imperial law of June 3^d anni 1900 concerning the inspection of the *slaughtering of animals* and the *view of meat* the official inspection of animals, to be slaughtered, before as well as after the slaughtering and the inspection of all meat imported from abroad was made obligatory in every case. Besides; for the prevention of *trichinosis* an examination of pork of every kind i. e. a microscopical examination of the meat was ordered in a great portion of Germany, apart from the ordinary examination.

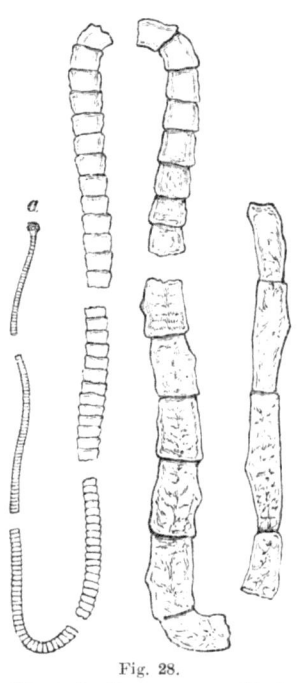

Fig. 28.
Pieces of a Tape-worm. *a.* Head.

§ 85. Preparation of meat. Boiled meat. Meat soup. Stewing; Baking and Roasting. The dangers, arising from animal and vegetable parasites are especially to be taken into consideration, if the meat is eaten more or less raw, e. g. as minced meat, smoked ham or as sausages. By thorough boiling or roasting the danger is generally obviated.

Boiled meat may possess an entirely different quality according to the mode of its preparation. If it is put on the fire in a pot filled with cold water, it becomes thoroughly saturated and loses a large proportion of its soluble constituents in the broth, particularly, if it has been cut previously into small pieces. This process of extraction is only interrupted or limited by increasing the heat to such a degree, that the albumin in the meat coagulates. If the meat is gradually raised to boil together with the water, we obtain a strong broth and a residue of meat, chiefly consisting of the insoluble tissues and the coagulated albumin. This "boiled out" *soup-meat* is not altogether valueless, but can still serve the purposes of nutrition on account of its albumin.

If on the other hand a somewhat larger piece of meat is placed in water at boiling point already, the albumin on the surface of the meat coagulates immediately, forming an insoluble layer which prevents the water from entering the interior of the meat and thus to transfer its soluble constituents to the broth. It is advisable to allow the water to act on it at the boiling point only for about five minutes and then to reduce the heat to 70 or 80° C. to prevent the meat to become too tough and difficult to digest through too great a shrinkage of its muscular tissue. By this process we obtain a weaker broth, but more nutritious meat.

The *broth*, obtained in boiling meat contains numerous flakes, consisting of the coagulated albumin of the meat and forming its most essential nutritive value. As these flakes are usually "skimmed off" in the process of cooking meat for the purpose of clarifying the broth and on account of their lesser value, the broth is generally poor in nutritive elements and insufficient as a means of subsistence; its value consists rather in a variety of salts and soluble, savoury substances, by means of which it stimulates the appetite and digestion.

The effect of *stewing*, or *slow roasting* in its juice is about the same as that of boiling meat; as by this process under the action of steam and a richer sauce the meat becomes more tender and juicy.

In roasting, the meat is exposed to the influence of a

great heat (with a layer of fat spread on the bottom of a pan), is repeatedly turned over, and to prevent it being burnt is being kept moist and is basted at intervals. In this way the meat gains in flavour and digestibility, without giving up a great quantity of its nutritive elements to the "gravy", which consists of the fat, the water and the juice of the meat. If the meat is *roasted* over an open fire, its salts and aromatic (savoury) substances are almost completely preserved.

§ 86. **Preserved meat.** As meat under ordinary circumstances quickly gets tainted and thus becomes unfit for food, several means and processes are used for the purpose of keeping it fresh. For instance; it is preserved in ice or, in cooling rooms, as at the lower temperature the germs of decomposition and mould do not usually develop; this however produces the inconvenience, that the meat so cooled easily becomes covered with moisture and thus receives the germs of decomposition and fermentation from the air. This disadvantage occurs in a much lesser degree by covering or enclosing the meat in canvass, hanging it up in a constant current of air and keeping it cool by proper contrivances. The meat thus treated is then not only cooled by the air, but also dried on the surface, and is protected against the ingress of germs from the air, both by the covering and by the dry layer, formed on the surface of the meat itself.

Other processes of preserving meet consist of cutting it in long, thin strips and *drying* it completely. These strips are then either preserved without further treatment, or cut into small pieces and then cooked and eaten.

A durable form of meet is *tinned meat*, which has acquired great popularity quite recently only. In its preparation the meat, either alone or with salt and fat added is exposed in tinned vessels for some time to a boiling heat or still higher temperature. The tins, being "soldered" hermetically, can generally be kept for a long period of time, without their contents losing its flavour. In some exceptional cases however it has been observed, that the tinned meat, probably from negligence in its preparation became tainted and otherwise dangerous to health; it is therefore advisable before cooking or eating tinned meat to examine it as to appearance and smell. Tins, whose contents are bad, can frequently be known by the cover having been forced up by the foul gases formed inside; the contents of such tins produce a splashing sound if shaken before opening. For a long time already it was known how to preserve meat in an edible condition by placing it in vinegar, milk and other fluids. Recently solutions of salicylic and boracic acids, sulphurous acid salts and other chemicals have been similarly used. But the employing of these preserving chemicals cannot be recommended from a sanitary point of view.

The processes of pickling and smoking meat are old and well-tried as successful. Pickling, so named after its inventor, the Dutchman Boeckels, pieces of meat, well rubbed with salt and salpetre are placed in casks in layers, one over the other. The salt removes the water from the meat, at the same time however likewise a portion of its nutritive elements, forming an uneatable brine. Pickled meat keeps well, but on account of the large quantity of salt which it contains, it has to be watered, before it can be eaten. After long continued use of it *scurvy*, a disease accompanied by inflammation and heavy bleeding of the mucous membrane of the mouth and the inner organs, frequently resulting in death, has been observed among sailors and soldiers. For the purpose of smoking, the meat, usually salted beforehand is hung in the smoke of burning or mouldering wood. It is thus deprived of water and penetrated partly by some ingredients of smoke, which are hostile to germs of disease (e. g. creasote and some volatile oils).

The so-called *quick-smoking* process consists in smearing the pieces of meat repeatedly at definite intervals with crude pyroxylic acid, which like smoke contains elements, hostile to decomposition, and afterwards hanging them up in the fresh air to dry.

§ 87. **Food, manufactured from meat.** Another method of preparing and preserving meat is the making of *sausages*. For this purpose the meat is cut small, mixed in different proportions with spices, sometimes also with an addition of bread, groats, flour etc. and then pressed into the guts of slaughtered animals. The sausages are either cooked, roasted, dried or smoked before being eaten; there is a great variety in this sausage making, and nowhere are there so many ways of making sausages as in Germany where the sausage enjoys a much greater popularity, than elsewhere. The nutritive

III. Food.

value and the taste as well as the digestibility of the sausage is often diminished by additions of little value; often the sausage is coloured artificially.

Sausage insufficiently boiled or smoked may cause injury to health on account of the animal- or vegetable parasites in the meat; justly dreaded is the so-called *"sausage poisoning"*, which sets in after partaking of tainted sausage. Of the different kinds of sausages the soft products which are either not sufficiently smoked or not smoked at all, are most easily exposed to decomposition.

Special articles of trade, which must be added to the animal food are *lard, bacon, and tallow*. The thick layer of fat under the skin of the pig forms *bacon*, which is either eaten boiled, but more usually salted or smoked as a nutriment, very rich in fat. The lard usually consumed, *pigs lard* is obtained from the intestines, but also from bacon by the process of melting.

It should be white and almost colourless, soft and melt at about 40^0 C. to a clear fluid and get solid again at about 26^0 C. It keeps best with the addition of some salt within cool places in covered jars of earthenware or porcelain, or in glass vessels, so as to prevent it from becoming rancid. A cheap substitute of pig's lard is sold under the name of *artificial eating fat*, a mixture of pig's lard with lard of less value and oil; by law it can be only sold under the above given name (cf. § 144).

The *tallow* of *beef* is firm and white, melts only at 42 to 44^0 C. and solidifies again at 34^0 C. It is less digestible than butter, which as food is also to be preferred to lard and bacon on account of its more savoury taste. Other ruminants also yield tallow (sheep's tallow), but these products are less often used as food than beef tallow.

Since about twenty years *meat extracts* have attained great importance. They are made by pressing or boiling of minced meat; the broth is then condensed by means of steam. The *meat extracts* are used in place of meat-broth by dissolving them in warm water; they are similar in nutritive value to meat broth. By mixing these meat extracts with flour, pulse, oats or potatoes meat or *soup tablets* are made as well as other durable forms of nourishment. They can also be baked with flour as *meat biscuits*.

Peptonized meat and jellies are also produced from meat. They contain besides the salts and savoury substances included in extract of meat, a portion of the albumin of the meat in a soluble form, and are easier digested than meat. But they have the drawback that they excite repugnance in many persons after a long-continued use.

§ 88. **Fishes.** Next to the flesh of land animals the flesh of fishes forms a pleasant change in our food; especially as it is similar in its nutritive value to the former and generally is as easily digested and assimilated as beef. However a distinction must be made between the lean and easily digestible fishes and the fatty, less digestible fishes. To the latter belong the salmon, herring, sprat, sardine, river-lamprey; to the former the pike, shellfish, sole etc. Sea-fishes contain considerable more salt than fresh-water fishes.

In fresh fish the gills are red, the eyes transparent and projecting; the flesh is firm, compact, elastic, smells freshly when the gills are opened, and possesses a white or reddish colour. Fish from swampy water possess less flavour and it is advisable to keep them in fresh water before killing. Owing to the presence of certain germs fish sometimes become luminous in the dark. But this luminousness disappears as soon as decomposition sets in, and is in no way a sign of an injurious quality to health.

But from other causes the eating of fish may sometimes cause injury to our health. Thus with raw or insufficiently boiled pike a germinal development of the so-called *"swiss tape-worm"* is received, which multiplies in the human intestines in the same manner as the worms of pork and beef. Then again, certain parts of some fishes contain poisonous substances, whose effects may be noticed for instance in *ba-belcholera*, i. e. a severe dysentery, which has been observed after the consumption of barbel. The tendency of fish to quick decomposition is also dangerous, and causes sometimes poisoning after the eating of fish, no longer fresh.

Attempts are made to keep fish fresh for a longer time by placing them on ice. Other devices for a similar purpose are drying (stock fish), salting (herrings and sardines), smoking (eels, flounders, red herrings), pickling, preserving in vinegar with spices (eels, herrings, anchovies), or preserving in oil (sardines).

III. Food.

By the perfecting of our means of transport it has be-become possible to send fish long distances, and thus make the rich treasures of the sea accessible to the inhabitants inland at a moderate price.

From the eggs (*roe*) of certain kinds of fish *caviare* is prepared by salting the roe. It affords a source of nourishment distinguished by a large proportion of albumin and fat and also savoury and stimulating to the appetite; on account of its relatively easy digestibility it is frequently given with success in many disorders of digestion and nutrition. In Russia caviare is obtained from the sturgeon, in Italy from the bull-head and tunny fish; in Norway from the codfish and mackerel; in England and Sweden from salmon and cod-fish; in Germany from the sturgeon and related kind of fishes. In the Dardanelles *fish-roe-cheese* is manufactured from the roe of many fishes by pressing and drying.

Train oil is obtained from the blubber of large sea-monsters by extraction. To commerce known is particularly the oil from whales, sharks, seals, sea-dogs and dolphins. Cod-liver-oil is manufactured from the livers of various fishes, that have been dried in the air and is used as an auxiliary nourishment as well as medicine for sick persons and for weak children.

§ 89. Crustaceae and shell-fish. Besides the fishes the water also shelters a number of "crustaceae" which serve as food for men. To these belong in the first class those crayfish, like river crayfish, lobsters, crabs, shrimps, whelks, whose flesh is estimated as savoury, but is not easily digested and is not procurable at all seasons of the year. Some people cannot digest crayfish at all, as skin eruptions develop themselves, which are similar to the blotches, caused by contact with nettles, and are therefore called "nettle rash".

To the creatures, living in water and used as human food also belong the mussles, commonly called shell-fish, viz.: oysters, edible mussels and cockless. The first named are mostly eaten raw, are easily digested, contain much albumin, also some fat, and are therefore useful not only as luxuries for healthy people, but as nourishment for very sick persons, who cannot digest any other meat. The other mussels are generally boiled before being eaten; as are also snails, which are relished in some districts as favourite food; especially the large vineyard snail.

As crayfish as well as shell fish quickly decompose after death, thus secreting poisonous substances, and as under certain conditions they also absorb poisonous impurities from the surrounding water, frequently *cases of poisoning* have been observed after eating them. Particularly mussels (moules) have frequently caused illnesses and the death of persons, since, after remainiag for fourteen days in stagnant water they develop poison in their liver; the poison however is said to disappear quickly, if they are placed in running water.

§ 90. Seasonings. Salt; vegetable acids; vinegar. Many of our foods require, in order to be eatable or palatable the addition of certain substances, which by their smell or taste stimulate the appetite and cause a more plentiful secretion of gastric juices; they also provide an agreable change in the form of the food, provided for us. As such additions we use particularly *spices* and *condiments*.

Among the seasonings *common salt* or chloride of sodium, a compound of the chemical elements chlorine and sodium occupies the first place, It is obtained either from rock-salt mines or from sea-water or from brine-springs. Common salt forms one of the indispensable necessaries of life; for it forms a constituent part of our body, is continuously being excreted from it and must therefore be constantly replaced. In cases of persons, who have exhausted their provision of salt, for instance in besieged fortresses or in long journeys in uninhabited countries a gnawing salt-hunger sets in.

Among the seasonings must be reckoned *sugar* (§ 71), table-oils (§ 66), various *vegetable acids* e. g. *citron* juice (lemon juice), citric acid and particularly *vinegar*. The vinegar used for the purpose of food is chiefly produced in acetic fermentation, which appears under the form of a special fermenting agent, the so-called "mother of vinegar" in alcoholic fluids (such as brandy, wine, beer and spirits diluted with water). Recently pyroxylic acid has been used in a purified form as seasoning; it is deposited by cooling the vapour, ascending from highly heated wood. The so-called „essence of vinegar" a fluid, very rich in acetic acid, and therefore very acrid, must be largely diluted, if its use is not to be followed by injurious consequences.

§ 91. Spices. While seasonings can still be regarded in some sense as a kind of food, the importance of *spices* consists especially in their savouriness and in their power of stimulating the digestion. They consist mostly of the roots, leaves, flowers, buds, kernels, husks, bulbs, seeds or fruits of certain plants, which on account of the ethereal oils, resin or other substances, they contain, possess a distinctive odour or flavour.

Many spice plants, as onions, garlic, mustard, radish, juniper, dill, caraway seed, aniseed, are produced in our own country; of foreign spices the principal kinds are: black and white pepper, bay-leaf, ginger, capers, clove, all-spice, stellated anise, nutmeg, saffron, vanille etc. Generally the spices, which we obtain from foreign countries have a high price, and are therefore often adulterated, especially, if sold in a ground-state.

III. Food.

§ 92. Refreshments. The refreshments (called sometimes "luxuries") stand nearest to *spices* in their importance as *human food* (§ 57). They are distinguished from them by being consumed, not as adjuncts to food, but independently of it in an unmixed state. We reckon among these refreshments alcoholic beverages, coffee, tea, cocoa and tobacco.

§ 93. Alcohol. Beverages, containing spirits of wine or alcohol are, when consumed moderately a valuable stimulant to digestion and are also used in many illnesses as a means for restoring strength and vigour. Immoderation in their use not only leads to drunkenness, but also to debility in the functions of the stomach and the bowels. After long continued indulgence in alcoholic beverages, severe diseases of the digestive organs, of the kidneys and the nervous system usually make their appearance. Therefore, confirmed drinkers frequently get disease of the brain, or meet with a premature death or tedious sickness; and they are less-able to overcome serious feverish illnesses than temperate persons.

Alcoholic liquors are obtained by allowing solutions of sugar to undergo fermentation under the influence of yeast. In this way besides alcohol, carbonic acid, fusel oil, glycerine, succinic acid as well as a series of other substances are formed. To the products of a fermentation of this kind belong wine, beer and brandy. While wine and beer can be consumed without any further special treatment, brandy can be obtained only by distillation from the fermented fluid (cf. § 47).

§ 94. Wine. Wine is obtained from grapes. The juice (must) is pressed out and collected in casks. Owing to the increase of the yeast fungi, already existing on the surface of the grapes, and therefore also existing in the juice of the grapes, fermentation sets in; and under its action the sugar of the grapes changes into alcohol and carbonic acid. A distinction is made between the *primary-* and the *after fermentation*. In the former the by far largest part of the sugar is decomposed with a strong formation of carbonic acid; in the latter the decomposition of the sugar remaining after the primary fermentation proceeds slowly with a weaker development of carbonic acid. At the same time the wine gains in bouquet and flavour. After some months the wine is transferred to vats, in which it further matures, till it is ready for bottling. In the production of red wine the skins and kernels of the red grapes are allowed to take part in the fermentation.

The so-called sweet wines (Malaga etc.) are obtained from the juice of particular grapes, grown especially in southern countries. New must of this kind yields in fermentation relatively large quantities of alcohol in proportion to its richness in sugar; some sugar however remains behind which does not take part in the fermentation and this imparts the sweetness to the wine.

Under unfavourable weather conditions, sufficient sugar is not formed in the grape to produce a wine, in which the acidity has been sufficiently overcome. If we wish to obtain under such circumstances wine rich in alcohol and less acid, sugar is added to the juice before fermentation. With the various artificial processess called Chaptalisation, Gallisation, Petionation etc. in most cases only an increase of the quantity of wine produced is intended. If the grapes, after the first extraction of juice are allowed to ferment with sugar, a weaker wine is obtained, which is mostly used as a domestic beverage. From raisins and water is obtained a beverage, called raisin wine. These wines and many other products are largely sold as pure wine. German wines contain from 7 to 12 per cent of their weight of alcohol; other foreign wines contain 18 per cent and even more.

A particular kind of wine is sparkling wine (Champagne), which was formerly made particularly in France, but at present is produced of excellent quality in Germany and other countries. In its production, new wine with added sugar is allowed to ferment in bottles, the tight corking of which prevents the escape of the carbonic acid produced. The sweetness and flavour of champagne are produced by the addition of *"liqueur"* (generally sugar syrup with brandy and aromatic ingredients) to the wine, after it has undergone fermentation. Recently champagnes made by dissolving carbon dioxyde under pressure in wine, mixed with sugar syrup and liqueur have been sold by the tradesmen.

In the manufacture of other vinous beverages, the so-called fruitwines, gooseberries, currants, bilberries, apples and pears are especially used: the juice of these berries is allowed to ferment with sugar and water added.

Wine belongs to the alcoholic beverages most beneficial to our bodies; all kinds of wine however are not of equal value, especially as regards their health giving effects. Sparkling and sweet wines are suitable for invalids, whose exhausted energies need to be recuperated as quickly as possible; white wines stimulate the motion of the intestines. Red wines are recommended for many digestive disorders and restrain a too violent motion of the intestines. Less valuable products, such as poor and raisin wine cannot serve as substitutes for wine in regard to its health-giving effects. Artificial wines may sometimes prove injurious to health on account of their ingredients. The labels, such as "Medicinal wine" or "Medicinal Tokay" often seen on bottles of wine are no guarantee that the products so designated are not injurious to health. On the contrary, just such wines as these are artificial mixtures. Home-made wines from reliable houses may often replace and often surpass foreign wines of uncertain source for use by patients.

§ 95. Beer.

Beer is less rich in alcohol, than wine. Of the materials, used in beer-brewing, viz.: *water, malt, hops* and *yeast* malt is the most important.

To prepare malt, barley-corn is allowed to germinate and thus the so-called *"diastase"* is developed, which afterwards changes the starch in the barley into sugar. The *"green malt"* so produced is then changed into *"kiln malt"* by drying; it is then bruised, after the germ is removed and is then finally mashed by mixing it thoroughly, first with tepid water and then with hot water inside a large vat. In this process malt-sugar, dextrine and other similar substances are produced. The fluid thus obtained, called *wort* is next boiled, whereby the operation of the *"diastase"* is finished; at the same time the hops are added: the latter give the beer its bitterness and flavour, and also make it lasting by destroying the decomposable substances. The fluid drained off from the insoluble portions of the malt (the grains) is then passed through cooling apparatus into the *fermenting cellars*, where yeast is added and fermentation allowed to proceed. The latter process, which takes place quicker or slower according to the temperature (*high* or *low fermentation*) changes the greater part of the sugar into alcohol and carbonic acid. The prepared beer is finally separated from the yeast and filled into casks, where it undergoes an "after-fermentation". Too extended after-fermentation makes the beer sour, muddy through the presence of yeast particles and injurious to our digestive organs.

Among the different kinds of beer we distinguish particularly between the *low-fermented* and the high-fermented strong beer, containing a considerable quantity of carbonic acid; to the latter class belongs the Berlin *Weissbier* (white, or pale beer). The colour of beer in general depends on the degree of heat, to which the malt has been kilned; however, pale beer may be coloured brown with sugar. Moreover, the quality of the beer depends on the manner of cooling, the length of the fermentation and especially on the composition of the "wort". The barley required for its manufacture is partly replaced by wheat in making pale ale, but it must be employed unmixed in brewing other beers. In some places other substances, such as rice, starch-sugar etc. are used in brewing, but the addition of them to "wort" is forbidden by Law in Bavaria.

The lighter German beers contain 3 to 4 per cent, export beer 4 to 5 per cent, "Weissbier" (Berlin pale beer) $1\frac{1}{2}$ to 3 per cent in weight of alcohol. The alcohol, contained in the stronger brewed English beer (porter, ale, stout), amounts up to 8 per cent. By a special proceeding a beverage, known as "*Malton wine*" has lately been manufactured from malt, which has undergone lactic fermentation, by the action of yeast. It contains 16 per cent, or even more (in volume) of alcohol.

Beer, brewed from pure ingredients is a very suitable refreshment for grown-up persons, and on account of the carbo-hydrates, phosphoric salts and other substances it contains is not void of nutritive value. Immoderate beer-drinking leads to the same injuries to health, as the abuse of other alcoholic beverages, and promotes the formation of fat in many persons. Strong brewed beer is considered an invigorating drink; thin beer i. e. poor in alcohol and particularly "Weissbier" form refreshing drinks, promoting digestion.

§ 96. Brandy. Liqueurs.

The various kinds of *brandy* form in different countries a popular refreshment for the poorer class of people instead of beer and wine.

In Germany *potato brandy* in particular enjoys a very extensive consumption. It is obtained by allowing the starch of potatos, that have been boiled in steam to change into sugar by mixing it with warm water and malt (cf. § 95); the mashed fluid is then fermented with yeast and subjected to destillation (cf. § 47). While the "*schlempe*" remains behind, the alcohol, with some impurities (aldehyd, fusel-oil etc.) passes into the distilling vessel and is either immediately sold as raw spirits, or is freed from its foreign elements by various refining processes and then used as refined spirit.

Other kinds of brandy are produced by the fermentation of the starch of rye, previously converted into sugar (corn brandy) or of wheat (whiskey) or of oats and maize. In France the beet-root juice, or the rich, sugar containing molasses extracted is used in the manufacture of spirits. By the fermentation of various fruits and roots, containing sugar we obtain *plum-brandy* (Slivovitza), *cherry-brandy*, *gin*, *hollands* and *Gentian*. *Rum* is made in the East Indies and the Antilles by fermentation and distillation of the juice of the sugar-cane; in the East Indies and Batavia "*arak*" is similarly made from rice mixed with palm-juice. Of all brandies the real, genuine *cognac*, obtained from wine by distillation is the most highly valued.

Next to brandy are to be classed the *liqueurs*, among which we know *Kuemmel*, Chartreuse, Benedictine, Danzig "*Goldwasser*", Curaçoa etc. All these liquids contain besides water and alcohol, smaller or larger quantities of sugar and flavouring substances, which are added partly as essential oils, partly as vegetable extracts. The so-called "*bitters*" are prepared without any sugar being added, from the extract of the bitter flavoured parts of plants with spirit and water.

The products of distillation are generally valued more highly than the drinking-brandy prepared by extraction from plants. The percertage of alcohol in these fluids varies very much. German drink brandy contains on the average 33, cogoac 40—50, rum 67—70, arak about 50 per cent alcohol of its weight.

The more valuable brandies are frequently *adulterated* by the addition of spirits of wine or other fluids. Particularly under the name of cognac, Nordhäuser etc. are sold mixtures of diluted alcohol with other sharply-flavoured liquids; the absence of spirits of wine is concealed by the addition of the so-called "brandy-acid" which is usually an extract of Spanish pepper. Sometimes poisonous colouring stuffs are used for the colouring of liqueurs and the aromatic substances replaced by worthless stuffs, injurious to health.

On account of its large percentage of alcohol, brandy possesses an importance for man's health quite different from wine and beer. Under certain circumstances the former stimulant is better suited than the latter for temporarily rallying the energies of a body, exhausted by illness or over-exertion. Moreover, many brandies, for instance good genuine *cognac* can be beneficially given in moderate quantities to invalids, weakened by long sufferings. On the other hand beverages of the brandy class lead far more easily to intoxication than beer or wine. Their natural impurities, such as aldehyde and fusel-oil and their adulterations produce injury to health, and if taken in large quantities at once, act as a sharp, and sometimes deadly poison (cf. § 236). If brandy or liqueurs are constantly drunk immoderately, bodily and mental ruin inevitably follows. The brandy-drinker usually loses strength and pleasure in work, impoverishes himself and family, because his means of subsistence disappears, falls a prey to other passions, becomes violent and very often a criminal. Frequently he becomes in the end a victim to *Delirium tremens*, if other diseases have not previously worn out his body, weakened by brandy. From statistics in the Prussian lunatic asylums during the years 1889 to 1891 it can be seen, that of the male lunatics, whose lunacy was neither innate (hereditary) nor merely due to disposition to lunacy in their family, *more than a third* of the number of cases of lunacy was due to diseases from *Alcoholism*, as far as a cause of the mental disease could be established at all. By an investigation of 32 837 criminals made in 1876 it was shown, that of 100 of these criminals 41.7 per cent were addicted to drink (drunkards). In countries, where drinking (the passion for drinking) is repressed by law and punished, a decrease in crime has been the consequence.

§ 97. **Coffee; tea, cocoa.** Besides alcoholic beverages *coffee*, *tea* and *cocoa* enjoy great popularity as refreshments. Coffee contains as its most important constituent "cafeïne", tea contains the similar theine and cocoa contains the closely related "theobromine". By means of these substances, these refreshments have an invigorating effect on the nervous system, the muscular activity and the circulation of the blood.

Coffee is the product of the coffee tree, which grows in tropical and sub-tropical countries, especially in Arabia, Persia, Abyssinia, Central- and South America especially Brazil, in Java and Sumatra and recently also in German East-Africa. On its branches grow cherry-like berries, each of which contains as kernel two coffee-beans. These beans are roasted, and reduced to powder by stamping or grinding. By pouring boiling water on them we prepare the hot watery infusion, known as coffee, which contains as its chief elements a volatile oil, tannic acid and "caffeine". For a cup of strong coffee about fifteen grammes of coffee beans are used, which contain on an average ¼ gramme of "caffeine"; all kinds of coffee do not however contain the same quantity of "caffeine".

Many persons, with whom coffee does not agree are fond of drinking instead infusions of home products, such as roasted chickory roots, beet, cereals, roasted malt, bread, figs, acorns etc.; which products are popular among the poorer classes on account of their cheapness. Such substitutes, which frequently contain tannin, but on account of their lack of "caffeine" do not possess the stimulating effect, are frequently but unfortunately used for the adulteration of genuine coffee, particularly when gronnd.

Tea is prepared by an infusion of boiling water or the boiling or roasted leaves of the tea plant, which is especially cultivated in China, but also in Japan, Corea, Java and other parts of Asia (notably at present in India). There exist two principal classes of tea, black and green tea; but their peculiarities do not arise from a difference in the plant, but from the mode of their preparation. The tea leaves contain generally one to two per cent of their weight "theine"; in addition tannic acid and very small quantities of gluten, starch and gum. The leaves of the willow-herb, of the sloe, of the strawberry of the wild rose as well as artificial colouring substances are used in the adulteration of tea; tea, that had been used already and then been dried is also sold as genuine tea. In Brasil and the neighbouring countries "*Mato*" or *Paraguay tea* is prepared from the dry leaves of the Maté; in its composition and effects it acts similar to asiatic tea. Among many nations a large number of other plants are used in the preparation of beverages, resembling tea.

Cocoa is obtained from the cocoa tree, a native of Central and South America and the West Indies, but which has also been transplanted into many other tropical countries (Cameroons). In the fleshy fruit, resembling our cucumbers lie the egg shaped seeds in rows; these are called cocoa-beans, and contain about 1½ per cent of their weight "theobromine", large quantities of starch, albuminous and glutinous substances and a fatty substance, known as cocoa butter. They are freed from the fleshy parts and roasted; in which process certain substances are formed, which give the peculiar smell and taste to cocoa; they are then broken up and ground. If a part of the fat is also removed from the beans, we obtain a non-oleaginous cocoa. If the shelled beans are ground between hot rollers the mass thus produced mixed with sugar, we obtain *chocolate*. These preparations, when boiled in hot water, generally with milk and sugar added, yield the beverages known as cocoa and chocolate. Chocolate is also eaten without any further preparation and is used for the preparation of many dainties in the kitchen and by the confectioner.

The starch, fat and albumin contained in cocoa give to the products of the cocoa-bean the properties of a food besides the qualities of refreshments. In particular cocoa prepared with milk and sugar can be recommended as a palatable and at the same time nourishing beverage. Cocoa and chocolate are preferable to tea and coffee in many respects;

they are better adapted for consumption, because strong tea and coffee, if used excessively for a long time, may cause injury to the nervous system, such as headache, palpitations of the heart and loss of sleep.

It must be regretted, that the products of the cocoa-bean are largely adulterated by worthless additions, such as animal or vegetable fat, the flour of cereals or pulse, acorns, chest nuts, heavy spar, plaster of Paris etc. Their value is also diminished by grinding the husks with the beans.

§ 98. **Tobacco.** To the refreshments we also add tobacco, which was originally brought from America, but is now grown also in other continents and particularly thrives in South Germany, France, Belgium and Hungary. It is used for smoking, snuffing and chewing.

In the manufacture of *smoking tobacco* the leaves of the tobacco plant are moistened with salt water and laid in heaps. After a kind of fermentation has been completed in them, they are dried, in order to be made into *cigars*, or to be rolled out as *roll tobacco* or to be cut fine. As the best smoking tobacco the products of the island of Cuba are sold by the name of Cuba or Havanna tobacco. *Snuff* derives its odour and pungency from repeated fermentations, often lasting for months, and from the addition of various odorous substances. *Chewing tobacco* consists of heavy, thick leaves, which are made into rolls. *Adulterations* of tobacco are frequent. For this purpose the leaves of other plants, or paper, coloured brown, are used; or genuine tobacco is steeped in certain liquids in order to give to it a distinct taste or odour.

Nicotine forms the most important constituent of tobacco, but the quantity of it in different kinds of tobacco varies very much. Taken in its purity this substance is extremely poisonous; but in tobacco smoke, or in snuffing or in chewing tobacco only very small quantities of nicotine pass into the human body. Its effects in the case of healthy grown-up men, inured to the use of tobacco are noticeable in a gentle stimulation or soothing of the nerves, and is aided by a certain satisfaction to the eye in looking at the wreaths of smoke, blown from the lips. In the case of young persons, unaccustomed to the use of tobacco, vomiting, pallor, headache, giddiness, faintness and other nervous troubles show themselves after the use of tobacco. After immoderate use of it symptoms of poisoning manifest themselves. In the case of habitual smokers sickness may also ensue after too excessive smoking, and with persons, who have for a very long time indulged too much in this pleasure, diseases of the nervous system and decrease of the eyesight are sometimes observed.

The excessive smoking of cigarettes from strong tobacco, rich in nicotine is particularly dangerous; which in burning in addition to the smoke of tobacco also develop the smoke of paper.

§ 99. Food utensils and food dishes (vessels). All food and all refreshments are, as a rule palatable and beneficial to our body only, when they are put before us pure and untainted. They can be wanting in these particulars, as has been pointed out above in individual cases, if their selection, preparation or storing have been carried out in a careless or improper manner, or if they are adulterated. Besides it may sometimes happen, that the good qualities of the food are injured by the use of improper utensils in their preparation or in cooking, or by faulty keeping by the buyer.

The eating, drinking and cooking utensils may be the cause of injuries to health, if the substance, of which they are made, contains poisonous metals, since the latter absorbed by foods containing acids or fats. Such injuries to health are for instance *lead poisoning*, which may arise from *lead compounds* used in the glasing of pottery, in the tinning of vessels or preserving tins, from the metal portions of beer, wine and vinegar pipes, of seltzerwater flasks, and children's bottles, and lastly from the tinfoil (which contains lead), used in packing, if these compounds pass into the food or refreshments. Even cleaning bottles with small shot has sometimes caused lead-poisoning, because through inattention single grains of shot remain behind in the bottle and are partly dissolved in the drink afterwards poured into it. For the prevention of such injuries to health an imperial Law was promulgated in the year 1887 (cf. § 144).

Cases of poisoning have been observed after using *copper*, *brass* or *German silver* utensils (forks, knives etc.), because *verdigris* had formed on them in damp air by the action of carbonic acid. If such vessels are to be used without danger they must always be scoured clean before use and thus freed from any *verdigris* that may be adhering to them. They should not be used in preparing acid foods. Boiled food should be removed from them before cooling, for the action of the air on the metal and the passage of the poison into the food is accomplished with great facility during cooling. The galvanizing of copper and brass and the electro-plating of German silver utensils affords a good safeguard against poisoning, but only, if the coating of tin or silver is complete and uninjured.

Zinc vessels are unsuitable for keeping milk, as when the milk turns sour, the zinc dissolves in it, and serious digestive disorders may ensue from its use; there is no objection however to the use of zinc vessels, which are well coated inside for the storage of water.

Iron vessels are usually provided with a coating of solder *(enamel)*, for otherwise they would give an inky taste and a discoloured appearance to food, stored or cooked in them. The enamel may become dangerous on its own account through containing too large a percentage of lead.

Aluminium and *nickel* vessels are also now employed for the storage and cooking of food. No grave objections have been raised against their use.

Sometimes food utensils are painted with injurious colours; for instance *green* bread or fruit baskets are sold, which contain arsenic in their colouring matter and hence may communicate poisonous properties to the contents of the basket.

Lastly; it is to be specially observed, that eating-utensils may *propagate infections diseases* if they have been used by persons afflicted with such maladies and are subsequently used by other persons without carrying out suitable precautions beforehand. If such vessels, after having been used by sick persons, are boiled for some time, or are thoroughly disinfected in such a manner, as a competent medical adviser prescribes, they lose their dangerous qualities. Moreover all vessels, used for cooking or storing food or refreshments must be first thoroughly cleansed, as the impurities, adhering to them, such as dust particles etc. can easily contain injurious substances.

§ 100. Storage of food. The *storage rooms for food* and refreshments ought to be dry, airy and of even temperature; i. e. they should be safeguarded from frost. Meat and meat, food are best hung free, so that the single pieces do not touch each other (cf. § 86). *Bulbous vegetables* may be kept in quantities in earth holes, lined with straw, or in boxes, filled with sand. In storing *potatoes*, it ought to be noted that the rotten ones should be removed at once, as otherwise the whole supply will become bad.

The ingress of *insects* is prevented by meat-safes or bell shaped wire grating. Large pieces of meat, ham etc. can be protected by covering them with linen bags. *Ice safes* must be carefully scoured with hot water and soda, since otherwise food stored in them acquires an unpleasant flavour. Strong *smelling food*, for instance cheese are to be kept apart from such food which absorbs odorous particles. As a rule we ought carefully avoid in storing everything which can injure the flavour, for the flavour stimulating the appetite is necessary for digestion and therefore is beneficial to the body from the point of view of health.

IV. Clothing.

§ 101. **Clothing as a protection against cooling.** The human body constantly gives off quantities of heat to the surrounding atmosphere, which quantities are greater, the lower the temperature of the air is. The *clothing* offers a protection against the cooling thus caused, which is specially notable in temperate and cold climates. Various *materials* are used in its manufacture, which are taken partly from the *animal kingdom*, as furs, leather, wool feathers, horsehair and silk; partly from the *vegetable kingdom*, as linen, cotton and india-rubber. The protection afforded to the body by such materials depends on their mode of *being woven* and their *heat conducting power*. Materials which conduct heat badly — that is, slowly absorb and slowly diffuse it — best counteract the effects of cold. It is of course not a matter of indifference, whether the body is surrounded by *a single layer* of clothing or with several garments, one laid on top of the other; the air between the different layers of clothing acts the same as a bad heat-conductor, separates the skin from the cold air round it and does not permit an immediate interchange of heat between them. For the same reason *porous material* on account of the air enclosed in its pores contributes more to the preservation of the heat of the body than thick material. This explains, that our hands and our feet get easily cold in winter, when enclosed in tight leather gloves or boots, which do not permit the formation of a warm layer of air between our skin and these articles of clothing. Polar animals are specially fitted for enduring severe cold, because

IV. Clothing.

they carry with them — the mammals in their furs, the birds in their feathers — and they are able to temporarily increase its volume by bristling their hair or ruffling their feathers.

Of the materials used for clothing, *woolen stuffs* afford a more effective protection against cold, on account of their greater porosity, than materials made from *cotton, silk* or *linen;* the *spongy rough washing leather* keeps the body warmer than smooth *patent-leather; furs* are more beneficial in proportion to the length and thickness of the hairs. All these materials use their capacity for maintaining the heat of the body, by storing up the air; if they loose their hairs or pile by much wearing, or if by taking up *dirt* and *dust* they are becoming less capable of storing air. Even the *dyeing* of clothing materials may injure their cold-resisting capacity, if the pores in the fabric are lessened in size by the colouring dye-stuff.

§ 102. **Clothing as a protection against dampness.** Besides the capacity of retaining air, many clothing materials are also capable of retaining moisture in their fibres and pores. They prevent in this way rain from penetrating to the skin, absorb the acqueous vapour from the atmosphere and the perspiration of the body and in this way *protect the surface of the body from dampness*. This advantage lasts however only so long, until a certain degree of saturation of the material is reached. Moisture, which exceeds this degree overflows the pores and gives a damp character to the material, which produces uncomfortable sensations on the surface of the skin. At the same time the evaporation of the surplus moisture causes a cooling, which is felt to be equally unpleasant and affords an occasion for colds.

Among our clothing materials *wool* absorbs moisture more slowly than *cotton, silk* or *linen*, moreover the last-named materials are very soon saturated with moisture, while the absorbent capacity of wool is far less limited. Furthermore silk, linen and cotton possess the unpleasant property of lying close to the skin when damp or wet, thereby producing the sensation of dampness on the surface of the body and favouring our catching cold; whereas wool, thanks to the elastic filaments, which give it its rough appearance lies even further from the skin, when thoroughly saturated, and allows a layer of air to continue as a safeguard against damp and cold. On the other hand, *wool* as a clothing material is not lacking in *certain injurious qualities*. Under certain conditions it promotes excessive perspiration, which may be weakening the body; it delays the evaporation of perspiration and permits in summer refreshing cooling less than other materials. And, as wool is generally relatively dearer, easily wears cut in washing and by the reception of dirt and dust acquires an untidy appearance more slowly than other materials, it is usually cleaned less frequently than others. Woolen clothes therefore contain often large quantities of dirt; these not only lessen its capacity for absorbing air and water by filling up the pores of the material, but may also cause direct injury to health. Lastly it must be mentioned that woollen underclothing sometimes causes severe irritation of the skin in persons not accustomed to it.

§ 103. **Selection of the material for clothing.** There is no clothing material to be preferred to others in every respect. Therefore in our choice we must pay attention to the *season of the year*, the *conditions of the weather*, the *occupation* and *state of health* of the person to be clothed; moreover materials for *underclothing* are to be selected differently from those for *outer clothing*.

In general wool is to be preferred, if it is intended to protect the body against frost, sudden cooling or wetting, while other materials may be freely selected as light clothing in warm, dry seasons of the year. Persons, who, in consequence of their occupation expose their bodies to the influence of the weather or become heated through muscular exertion and must then expose themselves to sudden cooling, for instance masons, sailors, pedestrians should wear woollen *underclothing;* but in summer they ought not to wear too thick materials, because the accumulation of heat produced by muscular labour becomes dangerous by prolonged prevention of cooling; it may even lead to sunstroke.

Woollen underclothing is especially suitable for persons, who are disposed to catch cold, particularly to troubles with their respiratory organs, rheumatism of the joints and the muscles.

Linen or *cotton* underclothing is recommended in occupations, which do not require any particular muscular effort, and are carried on in rooms of a pretty constant temperature. One advantage of such clothing is its lightness and its pleasant qualities after more frequent change of clothes.

The choice of materials for outer garments is almost exclusively regulated by the season of the year and the weather. In winter thick woollen stuffs are worn; in severe cold furs; in summer garments of linen, cotton and silk. Woollen materials, which have been made *waterproof* by particular processes i. e. whose fibres have been deprived of their power of absorbing water protect the body best from getting wet. These have the advantage over the *india-rubber* materials, used for the same purpose that they are pervious to air, and therefore allow evaporation of the moisture of the skin, without which unhealthy disorders of its functions may easily ensue.

§ 104. **Colour; shape and fastenings of garments.** In the choice *of garments* their *colour* also is not unimportant; because dark materials absorb the warm rays of the sun better than bright; therefore become easily warm in summer, and are to be preferred for winter use, while the latter are justly preferred in hot weather. We should also assure ourselves that no poisonous colours have been used in dyeing the materials selected.

The *manner in which the clothing is worn* is likewise not indifferent for our health. Our garments should neither interfere with the free movement of the body and its limbs, nor with breathing, digestion or the circulation of the blood. Oppressively tight fitting garments are to be avoided, because they interfere with circulation as well as with the functions of the skin by compressing the skin-glands, and they do not permit of the formation of a layer of air between the skin and the garment.

§ 105. **Clothing for the neck.** By tight clothing around the neck obstacles are placed in the way of our breathing, and to the reflux of the blood from the head and brain, which may give rise to choking, to congestion of the brain, heading and fainting. On the other hand loose clothing around the neck assists the secretions from the skin with advantage, as it favours an interchange between the outer fresh air and the air under the garments of the trunk. Hardy persons like sailors dispense without injury with any covering of the neck; anyone however less inured to the influence of the weather does well to protect the neck against sudden cooling by suitable covering. Young and healthy persons are to be warned however against effeminacy through wearing thick mufflers, fur collars etc.

B. The necessaries of life for the individual man.

§ 106. Constriction of the body by the clothing, or by the way of fastening it. The fastening of the trousers by a *belt* prevents the movements of the intestines necessary for digestion and may contribute to the formation of what are called *abdominal ruptures*.

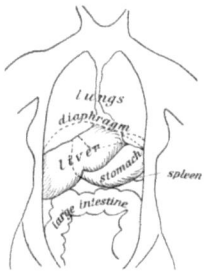

Fig. 29.
Position of the thoracic and abdominal intestines in the natural formation of the thorax.

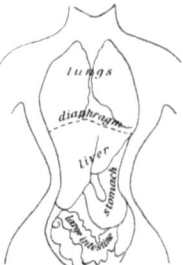

Fig. 30.
Position of the thoracic and abdominal intestines in malformation of the thorax by tight lacing.

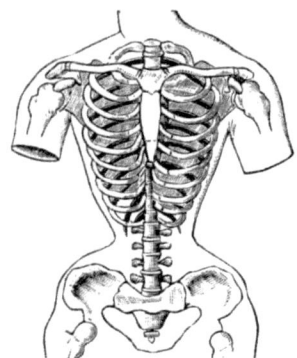

Fig. 31.
Malformation of the thorax through tight lacing.

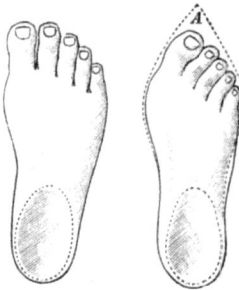

Fig. 32.
Malformation of the foot in a pointed shoe (A).

These begin as a rule gradually, when the intestines (on drawing a deep breath, or coughing, another point of expansion becomes impossible or difficult; force their way outwards by degrees as far as the abdomen as far as the skin between the muscular fibres and the sinews; usually in the neighbourhood of the pelvis or close beneath it, near the upper thigh (cf. § 7). In exceptional cases violent sudden shocks to the abdomen, as in jumping for instance can be the cause of rupture. This is in itself a troublesome malady and can moreover cause digestive disorders and severe indispositions in case it is not confined by a suitable appliance, a *truss*.

The improper use of *corsets* by women, who believe that they are beautifying their forms by tight lacing may cause injury to their health. For tight lacing not only affects injuriously breathing and digestion, but also leads to disturbances of the circulation, to changes in the position and malformation of the inner organs and may even cause deformities of the bones (Fig. 29 to 31). For the same reason warnings must be given against the use of rubber belts and the tying of petticoats (skirts) too tight.

§ 107. **Garters; Boots and shoes.** Tight *garters* prevent the circulation of the blood in the veins of the lower leg and foot and so cause the confinement of the blood to these limbs and the *swelling* of these *bloodvessels*, sometimes even so far, as to burst the veins and cause dangerous bleeding. In the neighbourhood of such swollen veins are often formed painful *ulcers*, which are difficult to heal. It has been therefore recommended not to fasten long stockings by means of tight garters, but by means of elastic bands, connected with the upper garments.

Particular attention must be paid to comfortably-fitting *boots*, which correspond to the natural shape of the foot. The shoe or boot should grasp the instep firmly, and not contract the heel too much, and leave sufficient space for free play of the toes, which at every step move forwards by the flattening of the arch (cf. § 11) of the foot beneath the weight of the body. In consequence of the different shape of the two feet the right shoe must be different from the left. The *stockings* or *wrappings round the feet* must not be creased and ought to be kept carefully clean on account of the vigorous and frequent action of the feet. *High heels* render walking and standing difficult, as the elevation of the heels occasions an uneven exertion of the sinews of the flexor and extensor muscles, thereby easily tiring the muscles of the lower leg, creating moreover a disproportionate distribution of the weight upon the foot, inasmuch as that portion of the weight of the body, which under ordinary circumstances rests on the heels is thrown too much on the ball of the foot. A *pointed shoe* contracts the toes, thereby causing a malformation of the foot (Fig. 32) and promotes the painful *ingrowing of the toe-*

nails into the soft tissues on the sides. The pressure of badly made shoes causes painful swellings, so-called *corns*, blisters and *bunions*.

All these evils, caused by defective shoes, even though they appear trifling in themselves lead to the mischief, that they prevent the persons, afflicted with them from taking part in those exercises in the open air, which health requires. If the feet are not washed frequently and carefully, painful inflammations may arise through the penetration of dirt into the sore spots which sometimes may have serious consequences in regard to the utility of the feet, or the life of the individual. For the avoidance of such dangers cleanliness is imperative especially for such persons, whose feet perspire easily and freely. Perspiration of the feet causes the accumulation of dirt and abrasions of the skin by means of the chemical decomposition which results therefrom, is easily perceived by its repulsive smell, and is the source of various diseases of the feet.

§ 108. **Covering of the head.** A heavy or unsuitable *covering for the head* causes a feeling of oppression, giddiness, headache, and contributes also to baldness, more especially, when it disturbs the airing of the skin of the head so covered by obstructing the free passage of air. The head-gear should therefore be light, should not press heavily on any part, and should either be made of porous material, or be provided with ventilating holes. In order to afford protection to the head and neck againt rain and the rays of the sun a broad brim is advantageous.

§ 109. **The Bed.** At night during our rest, while the clothing worn during the day is put aside, and exchanged for light night dresses, the bed affords protection against chills. On account of the proportionately smaller capacity of the body for evolving heat, when at rest thicker materials are selected for bed-covering than for clothing. For healthy grown-up persons *woollen* or *thickly-lined* blankets or counterpanes are however sufficient as *bed-covering*, and for *bed mattresses* full of pinegrass, shavings or horsehair or well stuffed with straw. Heavy feather beds render the passage of air between the surface of the skin and its surroundings difficult, and if they are used at bedding, they tend to make the body effeminate. They can be recommended only for children.

old men and invalids for whom a large amount of heat is necessary. For the sake of cleanliness the counterpane is supplied with a *cover* and the underbed with sheets from *linen* or *calico*, which can be easily washed or exchanged. By means of frequent and regular shaking and airing the bedding should be freed from the dust particles and skin excreta which accumulate in it. The frame of the bed in order to render the access of air easy, must be raised from the ground and is also to be kept carefully from vermin.

§ 110. **Cleanliness of clothing and bedding.** The *cleanliness* of *clothing* and *bedding* is of the very greatest importance for the preservation and furtherance of our health. As dirt prevents the access of air (§ 101), causes foul odours by decomposition and readily aids the germination of diseases, it should not be tolerated on our clothing; no more than on our skin (§§ 49, 50). Undercothing should therefore be frequently and thoroughly washed, and the outer garments should be daily brushed and shaken. The garments of others should never be worn without a thorough previous cleaning and linen should never be used, without a thorough previous washing.

V. The dwelling.

§ 111. **Purpose of the dwelling.** As a protection against the severity of the weather the dwelling serves in addition to our clothing. It not only affords us a shelter from rain, wind and cold but it is also a centre of family life, whose successful development forms the most reliable basis for the health of the people and for a strong orderly Commonwealth. The attainment of healthy and comfortable dwellings is one of the most important duties of public Hygiene.

A *healthy* and *comfortable* dwelling should be *roomy, warm, comfortable* and *dry*, and should neither harbour *foul air*, nor *dirt* nor *disease-germs*. The fulfilment of these conditions depends upon the building-ground, position, building-materials, roofing, interior structure, utilization of the dwelling-rooms, the arrangements for ventilation, heating, lighting and removal of refuse and lastly on the care and cleanliness of the inhabitants.

§ 112. **Subsoil and site of the house.** The *subsoil* of a dwelling-house should be dry and free from decomposing substances, so that moisture and unhealthy exhalations from the earth may not penetrate into it. A clean, firm, sandy soil on a somewhat elevated position, which at the same time is favourable to the flowing off of the water forms a suitable site for building a house. If water is met with at a small depth, it is necessary to drain it off by pipes. Where this is not possible it is advisable to line the foundation walls and basement of the building with suitable materials, such as asphalt or concrete, or to keep the water at a distance by so-called isolating walls. Such protecting walls to keep cellar-dwellings dry must be constructed of the most impenetrable stones and cement mortar; they must penetrate deeper into the ground than the foundations of the building, and be separated from them by an air space *several centimetres thick*.

Pollutions of the *building subsoil* must be removed by digging out the earth to a considerable depth and by replacing it with good sand. Filling up the subsoil with dirt and refuse is highly objectionable.

The ingress of air and light must not be impeded by the *position of the house*. A dwelling house open on all sides is therefore as a rule preferable to a house built in a narrow street, although a site, which is protected against cold north- and biting eastwinds offers other indisputable advantages.

§ 113. **Building-materials.** As building-materials for dwelling-houses we use wood, natural stone (especially sandstone, limestone, marble and granite) or bricks, formed of clay and burnt. As cement for binding stones *mortar* is generally used, a material, composed of lime, sand and water, which quickly solidifies, and should dry in not too long a period of time.

For judging building material from the point of view of health, its *porosity* and *dryness* ought to be of decisive value. By means of the pores of the walls a certain interchange takes place between the air of the house and the outer air. This so-called *natural* ventilation (airing) which proceeds without artificial means, such as opening of doors, windows or ventilators supplies the occupiers of the house with a portion of their air.

Porous building material is therefore preferred, especially because porous walls in summer protect the house from the direct summer heat and in cold weather best keep it warm; for the air enclosed in the pores prevents the same temperature existing inside and outside the house in the same way, as porous garments protect the body from chills (§ 101).

Of the building materials mentioned, limestone, wood, mortar, brick and sandstone possess more or less sufficient number of pores, which explains, why a wall, constructed of the latter stones always feels cold, unless directly heated by the sun. The above mentioned materials are therefore preferred for the walls of a *dwelling house*, whilst marble and granite are most employed for ornamental palaces and statues or other monumental buildings.

Besides the porosity the *dryness of the building material* guarantees the healthy character of the house. Moisture closes the pores and thus lessens the quantity of air contained in the walls, and reduces their heat-retaining capacity; at the same time its inevitable evaporation contributes to further cooling. A damp wall therefore always feels cold air usually emanates from buildings, which are not yet dried. Moreover moisture favours the development of various classes of fungi, such as "dry-rot", whereby the durability of woodwork is endangered, damp air is produced in the house and a mouldy smell generated. Such fungus growth also pass over to the house utensils, bread, and other victuals and destroy them; and it is not improbable, that the germs of many illnesses find in damp walls suitable conditions for their development and multiplication.

§ 114. **Drainage and drying of the House. The roof.** The healthy dryness of a house not merely depends on the quality of the building ground and materials, but essentially on the certainty and thoroughness, with which the drying of the rough structure is effected. Before a building can be regarded dry in a sufficient degree, the greater part of the water, introduced into the walls with the mortar, the quantity of which is estimated at about 85 000 litres for a middling sized town dwelling house, must be evaporated. This process is quickest effected by a strong current of air and is aided in cold or damp weather by good stoves and by opening the windows. Only when the drying has progressed sufficiently, should the shell of the house be plastered and further finished.[1]) Even a completed house requires thorough airing and drying, before it can be inhabited without injury to health.[2])

From a *later* injurious soaking of the house by the action of rain etc. the building is protected by plastering and painting, which at the same time gives to the house a more pleasant aspect. Lime is used for plastering dwelling rooms. Plaster of Paris is used for stucco work and combined with "water glass" for the manufacture of external water proof linings, cornices etc. Among the means for effecting this, whitewash offers least resistance and oil colours the greatest resistance to the flowing in of water. All these coverings of the walls gradually succumb to the effects of the air by crumbling; they become moist and the water permeates them; they must be therefore renovated from time to time.

To a great extent *the roof* of a building contributes a good deal to its dryness. Rain and snow should therefore nowhere in the roof find holes, but should be able to flow off freely over it and be quickly and completely carried off by pipes from the roof. As material for roofs in houses, the garrets of which are to be inhabited, tiles are especially suitable; for tiled roofs, which are laid upon rafters and joists, and are provided with a sufficient number of sheltered openings to insure a thorough ventilation of the lofts are the surest protection against dampness and cold. On the other hand, in rooms under slate and metal roofs the air is often close, in summer hot, and in winter difficult to heat. By their cheapness are recommended roofs from cardboard, strongly tarred over a framework of wooden spars, and roofs of so-called wood-cement, which consist of a thick mass upon a frame of boards, covered with fine sand or gravel.

§ 115. **The final touches on a house. Floors. Walls.** In order to maintain a sufficient intervening layer between the floor of an upper and the ceiling of a lower room, so as to deaden the sound, as also to promote the preservation of heat, it is usual to fill up this space with the lightest, the

---

[1]) According to the police regulations in Berlin of 1897 at least six weeks are necessary for this drying out.

[2]) According to the police regulations in Berlin — not before six months after the police certificate has been given, that the shell of the house is dry.

most porous, dryest and at the same time cheapest material. If such filling material is polluted with vegetable, or animal refuse, it may become the seat of foul-smelling decompositions, which allow repulsive and unhealthy odours to penetrate into the dwelling rooms; the use of contaminated filling-up material, particularly the use of building rubbish so freely employed formerly is to be avoided. Clean dry sand, coke-cinders, scoriae, peat or lime are suitable; still, even with these decomposable and putrid substances may penetrate through the joinings and cracks of the boards together with the sweepings, the scouring water and the dirt from the boots, if sufficient care is not taken to close the cracks in the floor. Where similar maladies reappear regularly in the same rooms during a long period of time, our thoughts will be turned to the possibility, that the germs of the disease have settled in the interstices of the floor, and can only be removed by renewing the filling it of the space between the two floors.

Wood is preferred as *flooring for dwelling rooms*, as it keeps them warm better than a stonefloor, it is used chiefly as flooring boards or parquetry. A coating of paint or wax increases the durability of wood flooring and increases the facility of cleaning it. Stone, cement and asphalt are more suitable for the floors of rooms, specially exposed to damp; for instance bathrooms and laundries. If the floor of cellars are formed of these materials (cf. § 112), it is usual to lay a wood floor over them, but so, that a layer of air remains between the two floors, which keeps the cellar warmer and protects it from foul air.

For the purpose of preserving the floor from dirt as well as to deaden noise and to increase the warmth and comfort of the rooms, they are usually covered with thick impenetrable stuffs, such as *carpets* of all kinds, or linoleum, manufactured with the help of cork. Carpets require to be frequently and thoroughly shaken, as they usually take up large quantities of dust, which may contain dangerous germs. Carpets should be entirely removed from sickrooms, because infectious germs adhere to them and are spread by them.

Wall-paper is usually found as a covering for the walls of dwelling-rooms instead of whitewash or paint, and as a rule no objection can be made to its use, as it gives the rooms a more pleasant appearance and protects the walls from damp and dust. On the other hand, wall-paper prepared from heavy materials is a great absorber of dust and can be cleaned only with great difficulty. The health of the occupiers of the rooms may be seriously endangered by wall-paper, coloured with poisonous substances, for instance arsenic.

§ 116. **Utilization of dwelling-rooms. Air-space. Plan of the dwelling.** Besides the character and structure of dwelling-rooms, the manner of their utilization is important for the health of the occupiers. The living of many persons in a narrow space injures the purity of the air, leads to the accumulation of dust and dirt and promotes the spread of infectious diseases. A dwelling that will answer the requirements of hygiene must therefore possess a certain spaciousness. Little value was formerly attached to that, and only in recent times the necessity of providing a definite amount of airroom for each occupier been recognised. As many large rooms, especially in old houses are insufficient for the air-requirements of the occupiers on account of their low ceilings, the Berlin police building regulations prohibit the building of dwelling rooms with a smaller height than two and a half metres. Still the wish of saving space in private dwelling oversteps sometimes the limit, asked by hygienic laws, and the air-space of 15 to 16 cubic metres allowed to each German soldier in his barrack room is not at the disposal of many people in their private houses.

Unfortunately, economy compels many people to combine in one bedroom, workroom, dwelling-room and kitchen. In such cases, the occupiers, as a safeguard for their health ought at least to air and clean the room as often as possible. Whoever is in a position to choose a larger dwelling should strictly maintain a *division between the dwelling-rooms* and those devoted to other purposes; in particular the bedrooms, the workrooms, in which relatively the largest part of the 24 hours of the day is spent, ought to be large, bright and airy.

§ 117. **Ventilation.** By sufficient space and a proper distribution of the particular rooms the quantity of air, necessary for human beings in a room is not yet sufficiently supplied; there is required a constant airing in addition; a *renewal* of the *air*, rendered impure by breathing and perspiration in closely inhabited rooms. The usual fresh appearance of country people occupied in the open air, as opposed to the ordinarily pale complexion of townspeople who spend the greater part of the day in closed rooms is a clear proof of the beneficial effect of pure air on the health of the human body. Moreover the effects of a defective air-supply are often noticed in the fainting of weakly persons in church, assembly halls and theatres.

The change of air, necessary in houses is supplied to a certain degree by natural ventilation (§ 113) but by far the largest part of the air, required by the occupiers must be provided by artificial ventilation.

The simplest contrivances for this purpose are large doors and windows, provided with fans and ventilating panes. The regular opening of the latter preserves the air supply with greatest certainty; however in rooms, occupied by several persons at the same time, this process is generally displeasing to some, and is often therefore neglected, through exaggerated precautions against draughts. In addition, in many houses there are air-passages leading from the outer walls of the house into the rooms, and opening, some just under the door,

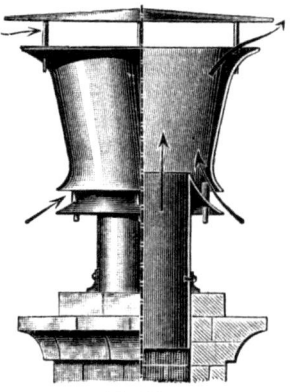

Fig. 33.
Chimney cap for ventilation after Wolpert.

and some close under the ceiling, so as to bring in the pure air below and carry out the foul air at the top. The so-called "ventilator wheels" which force the air into such passages and exhaust it from them are used for the same purpose. Lastly, the chimneys of the houses are fitted with special caps (Fig. 33) so that the wind, blowing through them, draws up and carries away the foul air. During winter the renewal of air is facilitated by the heating apparatus.

§ 118. Purpose of heating. Requisites of a heating apparatus. The protection, afforded to the house by walls, floor and roof is not sufficient in cold seasons to prevent the air in the house from becoming cold, and the occupiers from the effects of frost. We therefore try by heating the house to replace the heat, withdrawn from it by the winter frost; this is done partly by directly heating the air of the room by burning fuel; partly by introducing hot air, steam or water into the room.

The success of heating is greatly assisted by thick walls (cf. § 113) which conduct heat badly, as well as by tightly closing doors and windows, and particularly by double windows. The quantity of heat, given by various kinds of fuel is different; the heat, arising from combustion of coal gas is four times as great as that produced by burning wood; and between coal and wood, anthracite coal, charcoal, pitcoal and turf the capacity of giving off heat is in the scala just given.

The complete utilization of the heat, produced by the fuel depends essentially on the heating apparatus, as the latter may not only render the success of the heating doubtful, but also bring with it unhealthy consequences. A serviceable heating apparatus must give off sufficient heat in a season of strong frost and still must admit of being regulated so, as never to overheat rooms, requiring heat. It should further diffuse its heat uniformly, and not produce the state of things so frequently observed, that the floor remains cold, while the upper strata of the air in the warmed room are excessively hot. The fuel must be consumed as completely as possible in the heating apparatus, without leaving behind large quantities of ashes. The smoke and gases of combustion should not penetrate into the room, but have a good draught to carry them off. The air in the house should always possess a certain quantity of moisture (§ 35) and therefore should not be dried up too much by heating. Finally risks, arising from the use of the heating apparatus must be quite excluded.

The *injuries to health* arising from defective heating arrangements are manifold. Colds and chills frequently occur among the inhabitants of unequally heated rooms; smoke in the room causes irritation of the eyes and headache; the gases of combustion, particularly the dreaded fire-damp, whose most dangerous component is carbonic oxide gas, frequently produce fatal poisoning.

§ 119. Fireplaces and iron stoves. We distinguish between apparatus for *heating a single room* and contrivances for *heating an entire building.* (Local v. central heating.)

The simplest arrangement for single heating is the fireplace (Fig. 34) which communicates the heat directly from the open fire to the room to be heated, and carries off the gases of combustion up the flue without the help of a special *chimney*. As heating by means of fireplaces requires a relatively large quantity of fuel, only heats the rooms sufficiently in the neigh-

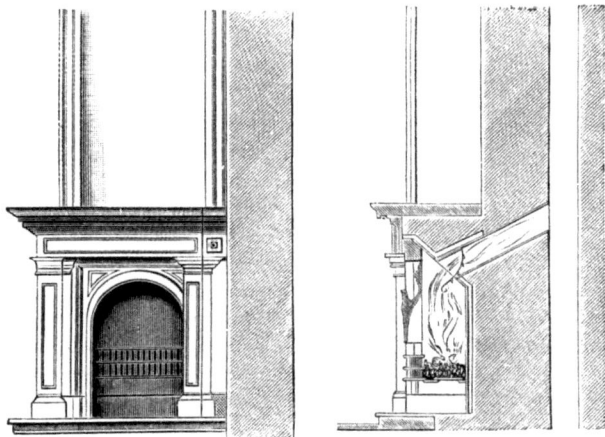

Fig. 34.
Fireplace in front.   Fireplace in vertical section.

bourhood of the fire, and does not prevent the smoke returning into the room, when the wind blows strong from certain directions, heating by *stoves* is universally preferred in Germany. In these the heat is first communicated to the heating surface, i. e. to the sides of the stove, and thence is distributed to the air of the room, to be heated. The remnants of the burnt heating material fall from the fireplace into an ashbox through a grating. Smoke and the gases of combustion escape through the stovepipe into the flue.

The value of a stove consists in its capacity for utilizing the heat of combustion. The more completely this is distributed to the heating surface, and the longer it is retained by the latter, the greater is the heating power of the stove.

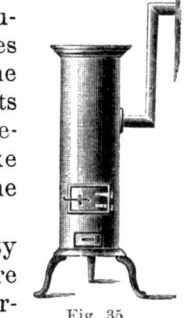

Fig. 35.
Cannon stove.

The simplest stove is the so-called "cannon stove", (Fig. 35) whose heating surface consists of a simple iron pipe, resembling a cannon. This class of stove heats itself and the surrounding air quickly, but cools just as quickly if the fire is about "going out", and therefore requires constant feeding with fuel. Moreover it easily gives off a burning smell, as the red hot iron pipe burns up the dust deposited on it from the surrounding air; besides the heat in its immediate neighbourhood is frequently unendurable, and lastly the flue usually is not quite tightly jointed, so as to prevent the entrance of smoke into the air of the room.

The last described evil was particularly dangerous to life, when *stove dampers* were used; therefore for many years stove dampers have been removed by order of the police. The closing of a damper in the stove-pipe just before its opening into the flue should prevent any escape of the heat of the stove. However it frequently forces the gases of combustion to find a passage into the room. Thus the above mentioned carbonic acid gas (§ 118) passes into the air of the room. This gas acts as a poison even in small quantities, and is all the more dangerous, because its presence is not detected by any peculiar smell.

A poisoning of the air by means of coal carbonic acid gas also took place in using the so-called *carbon-natron stoves*, a kind of iron stove, which was recommended for rooms without flues, because the coal, used in these stoves, called *pressed coal* developed little smoke.

§ 120. **Filled stoves; stoves with hoods.** It has been tried to remove the defects of the cannon stove by improvements. Thus, the *filled stove* was invented (Fig. 36), wherein the fuel for six, twelve, even twenty four hours is placed at the same time; in this way it gives out heat uninterruptedly for a long time, without needing refilling. The heat diffused by it can be increased or lessened by opening more or less a door, which is placed at the foot of the stove. By means of the *hooded stoves* a more uniform distribution of heat in the room is attained. The mantle (in iron stoves it consists of a cylinder of tin), surrounds the stove in such a fashion, that a free space, a few centimetres wide remains between the two, both above and below. The air in this space first becomes heated by the heating surface of the stove, and therefore lighter, than the air in the room; consequently it mounts upwards and issues from the top of the mantle, while fresh air enters below, is heated in its turn and carried out at the top. This circulation of the air in the room through the covered space, which has given these stoves the name of *"circulation stoves"* on the one hand renders possible the uniform heating of a large room, and on the other prevents the overheating of the portion of the room, lying nearest to the stove. If a pipe, provided with a movable damper is carried through the hooded space to conduct outer air into the latter, that is, supply fresh air as well as heat to the room. By such an arrangement the stove becomes a *ventilating stove*, serving for

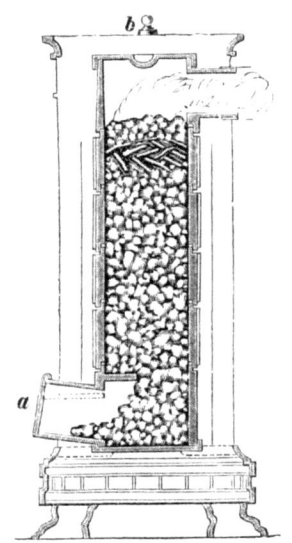

Fig. 36. Filled stove.
a. Door for regulating air draft. b. Aperture, closed by a cover.

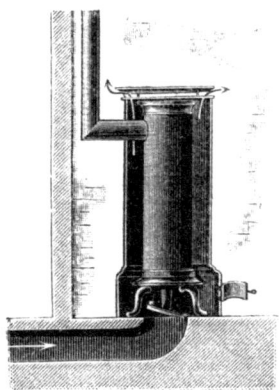

Fig. 37. Mantle stove.

ventilation as well as for heating. By placing a basin full of water near it, we can counteract the drying of the air, caused by the heat.

§ 121. **Earthenware stoves.** Metal stoves have the disadvantage, that their heating surfaces lose their heat as quickly as they acquire it, and hence require constant filling. The waste of fuel, thus caused is obviated successfully in the filled stove by the regulation of the air-supply, since the rapidity of combustion is reduced without interrupting the heating process. Still the *earthenware stove* is much more used in Germany than the filled stove (Fig. 38). In this, earthenware, which is a worse heat-conductor, than metal takes the place of the latter as the heating surface. Most earthenware stoves are in a sense mantle-stoves, for the heating surface is generally arranged in several *coils*, in order that the gases of combustion may give their heat as completely as possible to the stove before going up into the flue. As an earthenware stove heats only slowly, and loses its heat slowly, it always takes a longer time, than with a metal stove, before a room gets warm.

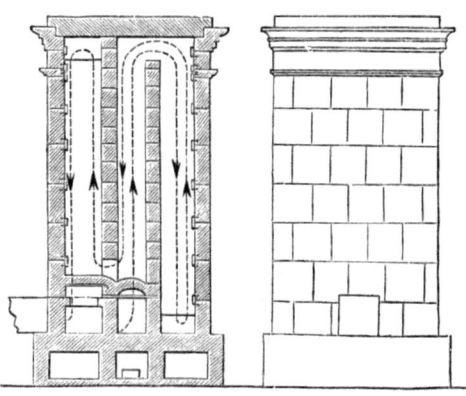

Fig. 38. *Earthenware stove.*
In section.   In front.

§ 122. **Collective heating by air, water or steam.** The inconvenience of heating single rooms inseparable from attending to numerous stoves in the same house is avoided by collective heating. In this process a large stove, situated on a ground floor, forms a source of heat for the entire house. From a hot-air chamber or a boiler heat is conveyed to all the rooms of the house by means of pipes, full of hot air, hot water or steam. While the hot-air pipes open freely in each room, and distribute the hot air directly to each, the water or steam remains in the pipes, which are arranged in numerous coils, in order to increase the heating surface, until reconveyed back to the boiler.

Collective heating has one advantage; i. e. the supply of heat to each room may be regulated, as required; in the case of hot air pipes, by valves, and in hot water or steampipes by cocks. An apparatus of this kind may be easily combined with ventilating arrangements, especially in the case of heating by air; for the air-supply for the heating chamber may be drawn direct from the outer air, before it is heated in the heating chamber and conducted into the individual rooms. On the other hand any disarrangement in the system of collective heating is very disagreably felt, because it is always perceptible in all the rooms, belonging to the same system. Hot water and steam sometimes produce unpleasant noises in the pipes and do not always afford sufficient heat, enough to warm the rooms; a steam heating apparatus is always liable to the danger of explosion through faulty construction or carelessness in management of the pipes. Hot-air pipes must be carefully kept free from dust in their interior; otherwise they contain easily charred dust, which fills the rooms with an unpleasant odour and produces a troublesome feeling of dryness on the mucous membrane of the respiratory organs. It is always useful to mix some steam with the hot air, so that the air does not enter too dry the rooms.

§ 123. **Protection of the house from heat.** By a properly arranged system of heating it is easy to obtain a comfortable temperature of about 18^0 C. in the dwelling rooms during the cold seasons. This temperature, as experience teaches us, is the most conducive to health, as it neither relaxes the body, nor does it produce the unpleasant sensation of rush of blood to the head, usually the result of a too high temperature.

The protection of the dwelling rooms from excessive heat in summer causes more considerable difficulties. *Thick walls* best keep a house cool. Where these cannot be constructed, it is well to procure a resting layer of air inside the walls as on the one hand air conducts the heat of the sun's rays absorbed by the outer wall of the house more slowly than stone, and on the other, as soon as it has become hot it ascends and conducts a part of the heat away from the house, when suitable openings for egress are made in the walls. Even the *colour* of a house is not without importance for keeping it cool, as the heat of the sun's rays is reflected from bright walls, but is absorbed by dark walls. *Metal roofs* become hot quicker and are better heat conductors than roofs of tiles, wood or straw. The rooms themselves are protected from the immediate effects of the sun's rays by *win-*

dow-curtains. Good *ventilating arrangements* contribute essentially to the cooling of a house, especially if the fresh air, conducted to the rooms is obtained from the shady side of the house.

§ 124. **Brightness. Natural lighting.** If *protection* from *summer-heat* is considered an advantage for a dwelling room, the *exclusion* of the *rays* of the sun is the greater disadvantage. Everybody has a longing for light; the healthy pursue their work more vigorously and cheerfully in a bright room, the invalid wants to have his bed drawn nearer to the window, in order to enjoy the light of the sun. Light, which illuminates the most remote corners of a room, impels us to cleanliness and destroys many of the minute bacilli, which are the cause of decomposition, putridity and disease. On the other hand dirt and dust easily accumulate in dark rooms; defective lighting depresses the mind, compels us to strain our eyes, and gradually injures our eyesight. Therefore; the dwelling should be accessible to daylight as much and as long as possible, though it may be advisable to cover the windows temporarily as long as they are exposed to the too glaring rays of the midsummer sun.

As a rule it is sufficient for the proper lighting of a room, if the total window-space amounts to a fifth or a sixth of its floor area; a wall in front of the window diminishes the entrance of light, and the distance between the wall and the house ought therefore to be at least equal to the height of the latter. The lighting is improved by bright wall-paint or light wall-paper in the room itself.

§ 125. **Artificial lighting. Candles. Oil- and Petroleum lamps.** As far as daylight is not sufficient, we want *artificial lighting*, either by the illuminating power of the flame, or by glow-heat. We value that class of lighting highest, which comes nearest to the light of the sun in strength, colour and uniformity, which does not produce too much heat, is unattended with any danger of explosion, and distributes least impurities to the air.

Candles manufactured from tallow, wax, stearine or paraffine afford an easy-flickering light, less endurable to the eye on account of the large admixture of yellow light; this light is not considered sufficiently strong to work by at the present time. Candles have the further disadvantage of giving off relatively large quantities of soot and of diffusing large quantities of noxious gases in the air of the room.

Lighting by means of lamps is more advantageous; in them various oily liquids are used as fuel for the flame. The essential parts of a modern lamp are. 1st The bowl for the oil, or other liquid to be burnt; 2^d the burner with the wick; 3^d the glass chimney and the shade. The wick, made from an absorbent material, hangs down into the bowl and sucks the liquid up to the outer edge of the burner, where it is consumed. The flame receives the air, necessary for combustion through lateral openings in the burner; it is protected from draughts by the chimney, and flickering is thus avoided. The regulation of the supply of air effects complete combustion and thus increase the brightness of the flame and at the same time lessens the deposition of soot and the production of noxious gases. The shade lessens the light which is too glaring for the eyes and if manufactured in the usual white colour suitable manner.

As an illuminant in lamps *petroleum* is now much employed; as compared with the rape seed oil, formerly much used, it gives a brighter light even with quite simple lamps. Petroleum is found in certain strata of the earth, where it has been formed by decomposition of débris from the vegetable and the animal kingdoms; it is subjected to a refining process before use, in order to free it from substances, liable to explode easily. However well refined, petroleum is a very inflammable fluid, and easily liable to catch fire; its careless storage or use has led to many accidents (§ 144).

Alcohol has also been used for lighting purposes.

§ 126. Gas lighting. Electric light. Brightness, steadiness and ease in manipulation are indisputable advantages of gaslight. The illuminating gas, manufactured in the gasworks from coal, by raising it to an intense heat in airtight vessels and afterwards purified, enters directly from the pipes into the burners, and is consumed in them without any smell and with a pleasant flame, whose brightness depends on the class of burner used.

Among the latter, the divided burner, made of soap-stone, which causes the gas to issue through a slit, and the Argand burner, in which the gas escapes from a soap-stone ring, pierced by numerous small holes are preferable to the single and double burners, the apertures of which do not allow a sufficient quantity of gas to pass through them.

124   B. The necessaries of life for the individual man.

Recently the incandescent light is largely used. It is produced by allowing a substance, composed of fire-proof materials to be raised to a white heat by a gas-jet. This mode of lighting consumes only a moderate quantity of gas and gives a very bright light without producing as much heat as an ordinary gas-flame. An important advantage for our health is the relatively small production of gases of combustion.

The use of gas for lighting purposes brings in its train the disadvantage, that the heat of a room so lighted often increases to an unbearable degree, and may cause headache as well as fainting. If moreover the gas becomes mixed with the air, which we breathe, it may endanger our health and life by its poisonous and explosive qualities. Such occurrences are sometimes observed in the case of leakages from underground pipes, particularly in basements, whose temperature causes a draft of air, which draws in the gas with it. In other cases, defects in the pipes within the houses, or careless turning on of gas-jets, which have not been turned off before, leads to injuries to health. Fortunately the peculiar smell of gas quickly directs the attention of persons present to the danger, which is obviated, by turning it off and thoroughly airing the room. Nobody should ever enter a room with a naked light, where there is a smell of gas.

On account of its high illuminating power acetylene gas alone or mixed with other gases has recently been much used for lighting. The electric light is also used as an illuminant. There are two kinds of electric light — the arc and the incandescent. The former is produced by passing an electric current between two carbon points, thus forming an arc of light; it owes however its great illuminating power essentially to particles of carbon raised to a white heat, which are detached by the current. In the incandescent light a carbonized platinum wire, enclosed in a vacuous glass globe is raised to white heat by the electric current. The electric light is steady and by proper shading agreable to the eyes; it produces but little heat, no soot or gases of combustion.

§ 127. **Protection of the eyes by shades.** With every class of light, the eye must be protected from too glaring and too direct rays of light; where the lamp-globe is not sufficient for this purpose, too bright light is moderated by various means (lamp-shades). Lamp shades of metal, which are glaringly white inside are injurious to the eye; they should therefore be used only, when the eye is removed from the direct action of the reflected rays, or when the purpose is to throw the light to a distance.

§ 128. Cleanliness in the dwelling. Removal of refuse.
A house, which is to serve as a wholesome abode for man requires *cleanliness* above all things. Dust, dirt, bad smells, foul air etc. have been already indicated several time in the preceding pages as enemies to health (cf. § 49). Their prevention and removal from the house is a duty imposed by the fundamental laws of hygiene.

For this purpose regular dusting, sweeping and scouring are not sufficient; there is required in addition careful removal of sweepings, domestic refuse and human excreta from the dwelling, the house and its neighbourhood.

Sweepings, house and kitchen refuse would be most reliably removed by burning; this modus however is difficult on account of the large admixture of incombustible material, which could be eliminated only at very great expense. It is usual to collect such refuse in boxes, or in other receptacles and to have them carted away from time to time. If the emptying of these receptacles is not done frequently and carefully enough, deleterious gases are diffused from the garbage, which are objectionable on account of their smell, and pollute the air in the house and its neighbourhood.

§ 129. Removal of human excreta. *Human excreta* have always been quickly removed from the dwellings on account of their repulsive appearance and smell and mostly emptied into pits, where the fluid constituents percolate into the soil, and the solid matter gets decomposed and dissolved.

Such *cesspools*, which even at the present time are frequently met with in the country not only make their presence felt far and wide by their unpleasant odour, but also contaminate the ground and the water of neighbouring wells to a considerable extent and can thus cause the spread of dangerous diseases (cf. § 44). By an airtight covering of the cesspool, as well as by lining its sides with masonry these inconveniences are not removed with certainty; even the thickest materials cannot resist permanently the action of the liquid excreta. Still, the pollution may be avoided for a longer period of time by double walls of cement, the space between which is filled with an impervious layer of clay, assuming that the contents of the pit are frequently removed by pumping or thorough cleaning. Better reliance for the removal of human excreta can be placed on the system of *pails* or on the *water carrying off* plan *(Schwemmcanal-System)*. In the former the human excreta are conveyed directly by outfall pipes into hermetically closed barrel-shaped reservoirs, which are carted away from time to time and replaced by similar empty tuns. In the water-carriage system. the outfall pipes open into subterranean pipes, in which the excreta are washed away by a flow of water conducted into them (cf. § 136, 137).

The *closet arrangements* for the first reception of the excreta (Fig. 39) should be placed in a space in the house, not too narrow, and as isolated as possible. This room should be well lit, to facilitate cleaning and should be kept free from smell by a thorough ventilation.

Where the excreta from the closet do not fall directly into the main sewer bad smells are prevented, by frequently supplying the collecting buckets with peat mould or other disinfectants and frequently emptying and cleaning them. Outfall pipes should possess a contrivance for preventing the return of foully smelling and unhealthy gases into the closet. A suitable construction of this kind is the much-used *syphon trap*, which provides together with constant flushing of the closet, that the outfall pipe of the pan projects in a $\sim$ shaped bend to meet the soil-pipe. The water collecting a fresh in this bend, at every flushing, separates the air in the closet-

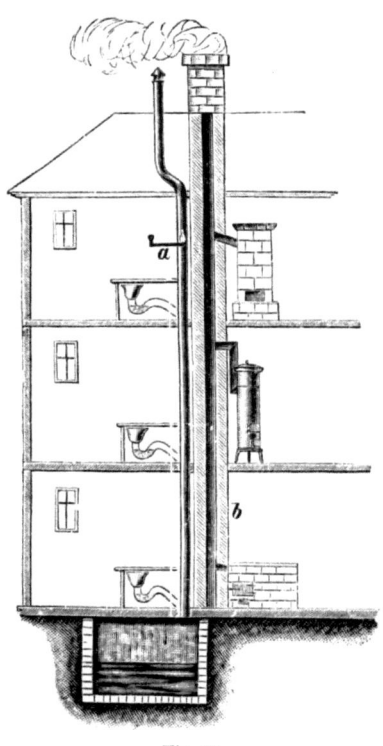

Fig. 39.
Closet arrangements in a dwelling-house.
a. Flame to attract air. *b*. Flue.

pan securely from that in the soil-pipe. The soil-pipe itself is continued upwards above the level of the roof, so that the gases contained in it, may escape into the open air. To that effect the air in the soil-pipe is sometimes heated, either by a flame burning in it, or by a neighbouring flue, and so caused to ascend. The soil-pipe thus serves at the same time as a ventilator of the cesspool, bucket, or outfall-pipe, the foul smells of which need not be drawn away by special ventilating pipes.

§ 130. **Hight of the dwelling. Attics and cellar dwellings (basements).** Important for the healthy condition of the human dwelling is its *height* within the house. Lofty dwellings compel to frequent ascents of the stairs, an effort which is not injurious to the healthy, but is often prejudicial to old and weak persons. The *attics* and *basement dwelling-rooms* must be considered also from a sanitary point of view with regard to their loftiness. In planning these dwellings it is frequently difficult to provide for sufficient air-space and proper ventilation; it is especially difficult to avoid on the one hand to have the attics more exposed to the summer heat and winter cold than the other apartments and on the other hand allowing the moisture of the earth and the exhalations of neighbouring dustbins and cesspools to penetrate into the basement story. In the basement story the lighting, as a rule, leaves much to be desired.

According to the building regulations in Berlin the floor of a dwelling room must not lie deeper than half a metre below the soil; only in the case, when a trench for light — the width of which must at least be one metre — has been constructed, whose depth is 15 cm lower than the floor of the adjoin room, a dwelling-room may be constructed as deep as one metre under the soil of the earth. The floor of such rooms must be however at least 0.4 higher than the groundwater at high-water level, and must have a tight unpermeable flooring. The sidewalls must be secured against dampness by isolating layers (cf. § 112), besides all other reliable means must be used for making such rooms absolutely secure against dampness. Attics can be used as dwelling rooms only, when not more than four floors below them are inhabited; they must not be higher than 18 m above the pavement; they must get air and light direct from the street, or from the courtyard, and they must be separated by means of fireproof walls from the adjoining parts of the roof or the garrets.

§ 131. **Articles for use in the dwellings.** With regard to the *articles*, necessary *for use in* the *house* and the *interior decoration* of the *dwelling-rooms* it must be pointed out, that furniture, carpets, curtains and other articles of furniture sometimes contain poisonous substances. Mostly these are colouring substances with poisonous metallic salts, especially arsenical dyes, which may be injurious to health. In the German Empire a law was promulgated on July 5th 1887, which regulates the trade with colouring substances for use in dwellings etc. It is advisable in buying toys, clothes, carpets, wallpaper etc. to have them examined for arsenic.

VI. Exercise and Recreation.

§ 132. **Exercise and recreation.** To the necessaries of man's life belongs also regular exercise. A sluggish body suffers injury to his health even under careful treatment and the lassitude, caused by inactivity easily leads to excesses, injurious to morals and health, the results of which are dipsomania and other vices. On the other hand body and mind require regular recreation and rest after labour, in order that their capacity for work and endurance may not suffer an injury; lest excessive irritability, relaxation, loss of sleep, headache and premature decay of the mental faculties ensue. The care of the health requires a just balance between activity and recreation, for which however general precepts cannot be established, since the working capacity and need of recreation are different for every individual. Above all is important for health *the way* in which the hours, given to rest besides sleep are made use of.

Intellectual stimulation on one hand, enjoyment of the beauties of nature on the other hand ought to fill out the time of recreation of every cultured person. Those whose calling compels them to undergo bodily exertion and exercise in the open air should rest the body during their leisure hours, and should seek recreation particularly in intellectual stimulation, viz. in enlightened discussion, in reading useful books or in contemplation of works of art or in the enjoyment of good music. On the other hand, he who is mentally occupied, and must spend his hours of work standing or sitting in closed rooms, should seek action for his body in his leisure hours by suitable bodily exercise, such as gymnastics, sculling, riding for the purpose of strengthening his muscles and by staying in the fresh open air should procure fresh, pure air for his lungs. But where bodily deformity or disease have

VI. Exercise and Recreation.

already injured the health, medical advice must indicate the manner, in which the leisure hours ought to be occupied most beneficially.

Social intercourse also affords a congenial recreation not injurious to health, when confined within proper limits. The exchange of thoughts with other men stimulates the mind advantageously; the communication of our feelings and experiences is a necessity for most people and requires social conversation as well as proper interest in the pursuits of our fellow-men. Only when social intercourse is joined to excessive bodily pleasures, when passions are thereby aroused and the body deprived of necessary sleep (in gambling) does it become as injurious as too much exercise of the body; for it injures our capacity for work, makes men disinclined for labour, and leads to premature exhaustion of the body and mind.

To spend the hours of recreation regularly in visits to badly ventilated taverns, full of tobacco smoke is not only injurious to the health, but very often to the pecuniary circumstance of the individual; still more injurious is the liberal consumption of alcoholic drinks, which usually accompanies (cf. § 93 and 96) it; but most ruinous of all is the excessive indulgence, which leads to the paths of licentiousness and vice.

C. Man in his relation to society.

§ 133. Communities. Public Hygiene. In the present state of society the individual has often to rely on the assistance of his fellowmen for the supply of the necessaries of his life. The success of the preparation of good and savoury food, of the making of suitable clothing and of the building of healthy and comfortable dwelling-houses is only assured by the united exertions and work of several persons. The more perfectly agriculture, handicrafts and other industries even art and science are able to satisfy our multifarious wants; the more the individual is compelled to devote his strength to a particular department or business and to adapt his work to the exigencies of a single pursuit; so much more he needs the cooperation of others for the supply of necessaries of his own existence.

This circumstance and the knowledge that in a community we increase our power of battling against animals and hostile fellow-men have caused families, tribes, clans and peoples to unite together, to form settlements in common, to create states, to seek mutual trade relations and to exchange those commodities, which are necessary for the wants of human life.

If therefore the union of men facilitates the preparation of the means for the preservation of life and health, it carries with it however on the other hand some evils, which are prejudicial to health. The perception and removal of such evils as well, as the improvement of institutions for the furtherance of the health of the people are the aim of public *Hygiene;* it is one of the most important and most beneficial problems and tasks of the administration of every country.

I. Settlements.

§ 134. Importance of settlements for health. The drawing nearer together of men to one another, the instinct of "gregariousness" have contributed to those common settlements, which are scattered all over the world as groups of houses, or in the shape of hamlets, boroughs, villages, small and big towns. In every one of these settlements the inhabitants are subject to certain influences, which are important for their health. These arise from the position of the locality, the character of the soil, the removal of refuse, dirt and garbage, the water supply, the extent and the architecture of the settlement and its laying out, the nature of crafts and industries; the wealth and degree of culture of the inhabitants, the supervision of the buying and selling of provisions, the care of the poor and sick people, the institutions for the burial of the dead etc.

§ 135. The Locality. For the purpose of judging the situation and locality of a settlement the same rules are applicable from a hygienic point of view, as for a dwelling house (cf. § 112); it is however as a rule easier to the larger number of people who are living in a community to remove injurious nuisances, than their removal would be to a single individual. The community succeeds better by clearing the ground, by levelling the soil, by blasting rocks etc. in obtaining a better access to fresh air; by the making of drains, ditches and canals, by the deepening and enlarging of running waters to free the soil from dampnes and to dry up morasses which experience has taught us to regard as nurseries of feverish illnesses.

§ 136. The removal of refuse in settlements. To keep the soil and the water clean requires in every communtity (settlement) particular care, as an injurious accumulation of garbage and excreta is caused by the living together in common of many people. How quickly this refuse accumulates is proved by the fact, that according to the experience in large communities each adult produces annually on an average 34 kg of excreta, 34 kg of urine, 110 kg of solid kitchen refuse sweepings and ashes, as well as 36 000 kg of waste water. It is therefore the duty of the communal authorities to superintend the removal of such large quantities of refuse and to regulate this work in such a manner, that the indifference or negligence of the individual may not cause injury to the community.

As regards the removal of garbage we have to consider particularly the cartage, the draining and the flushing.

Cartage is principally made use of, where the removal of dry refuse and of the human excreta, collected in pails and cesspools is concerned. The execution of this work in small communities is left to private individuals, while in larger settlements it becomes the work of a contractor. The removal is best done during the hours of night in the most inconspicuous manner. The tanks or other vessels used for the removal must be air-tight and water-tight to prevent contamination of the air and the soil.

Through *simple drainage* the water used in cooking and washing should be first carried off; the urine of men and animals is often carried off in the same manner, being partly received separately (in chamber vessels, urinals) and partly segregated from the solid excreta by special contrivances in the cesspools and dungheaps. For the drainage of water, subterranean, closely fitting pipes and sewers are better than the open drains and sinks, still in use in some small communities, as the filthy contents of the latter easily become stagnant, overflow and contaminate the soil.

In many larger towns and in most capital towns (Großstädten) the solid and the liquid refuse, exclusive of the *müll* (dry excreta) is usually carried off together by means of flushing through tightly fitting pipes in subterranean sewers. The further removal is facilitated by a sufficient slope of the sewers, by being mixed with the entire liquid refuse and by flushing, which process already begins in the water-closets. The rainwater is also generally permitted to run into the sewers, but in such a case it is necessary to retain the coarser street-refuse by means of so-called gullies from the places where the rainwater flows into the sewers.

The foul, ill-smelling and unhealthy sewer gases must be prevented from re-entering into the houses by means of Siphons (§ 119) in the closets and gullies.

To prevent flooding of the sewers by heavy rainfalls and for the prevention of floods special danger valves must be constructed, through which a portion of the too much swollen contents of the sewers can be discharged for some time.

§ 137. **The final destruction of refuse.** The final destruction of refuse causes no less difficulty than its removal. It is only facilitated by the fact that these masses can be used for manuring the soil, as they contain the materials for the cultivation of the crops, and because they are therefore useful to the agriculturist. For a long time already serious attention has been directed to finding a modus of transforming the refuse by suitable treatment into a form, in which it could be easily despatched and preserved for a long time. Either they tried to defer decomposition by collecting the solid parts separately and mixing them with dry deodorizing substances, as for instance turf-mould, or the refuse was worked into manure-powder (poudrette) at the same time destroying the germs of illness and decomposition. These two procedures, whose more extensive application remains perhaps reserved for a future time have not yet been hitherto much used. In many towns, villages and industrial establisments especially however in the capitals it is found more convenient to get rid of the refuse by some other means; it is usual to treat the different kinds of refuse in different ways.

The *dry house refuse* (Müll) is burnt in some places — for instance in many English towns — thus furnishing heat for using machinery. In Germany this procedure is not much used; they prefer to collect the refuse on remote open places and to leave it there to be decomposed, although it is not easy to find for a length of time sufficient space for the enormous quantities of refuse (Müll), which for instance in Berlin according to an authoritative estimate amounts annually to 700 000 cbm and requires 233 000 cartloads for its removal. Under certain circumstances moorland is a suitable place for shooting rubbish; for it gains in solidity by the closely parched solid parts of the refuse and thus can be more easily reclaimed for cultivation.

The contents of *closet tanks, cesspools and flushing sewers* can be got rid of in the simplest manner by emptying them into *running streams, or other water-courses*. This procedure however deprives the agriculturists of large masses of valuable manure and easily produces contamination of the water, which may become highly injurious to the health of the inhabitants especially in places, where the volume of water in the stream is not large, or where by a strong current the quick removal of the refuse which is introduced into the water cannot be secured (cf. § 45). For these reasons the contents of the closet tanks and cesspools are as a rule used immediately as manure, or the refuse in the sewers is subjected before being emptied into an open stream to special treatment, by which the substances, valuable for agriculture are retained and those injurious to health are made innocuous.

A treatment of this nature is known as the *clearing process*. The contents of the sewers are first collected for the purpose of clearing in large basins, as the elements of the refuse separate in consequence of their specific gravity being different. This classification (precipitation) can be promoted by substances which act chemically or physically or by mechanical contrivances, by some of these procedures germs of disease are also destroyed. Then the clear fluid is let run off into a stream, while the residue at the bottom is used for manure or otherwise.

Where the soil is suitable, the irrigation process proved to be very satisfactory, the sewer waters are allowed to flow over and to percolate into a field, which is somewhat sloping downwards, which lies low and is well-drained, the best is sandy soil. The sewage elements are thus retained in the soil, where beside mechanical filtration, chemical changes and a process of decomposition take place. The filtered water, freed from the refuse matter is conveyed by means of drainpipes into a running stream of water. By cultivation of an irrigated field with grain, vegetables or any other useful garden plants the innoxiousness (decomposition) of the refuse is hastened and at the same time its value as manure increases.

One disadvantage of the irrigated fields is, that during a sharp frost in winter the conducted sewer-water does not sink into the frozen ground, but seeks another exit over the surface or in the deep furrows of the soil, and thus flows in a contaminated state into the water-course. In time of frost the irrigating waters are therefore caught in large catchment-basins, in which they gradually sink into the ground.

§ 138. **Removal of waste water from factories.** Special attention must be paid to the removal of waste water from industrial works and factories. Many such places, for instance slaughter houses, glue-manufactories, paper-mills discharge refuse, which develop foul odours by reason of the large quantity of putrescent substances, they contain; with the refuse of chemical factories very often even poisonous substances are discharged; and to the refuse of slaughterhouses, tanneries etc. sometimes dangerous germs of disease adhere (for instance of anthrax etc.). The directors of such factories must therefore be compelled to make the refuse from their factories innocuous and to remove them entirely; for this purpose similar arrangements have to be made as for the removal of refuse from dwellings.

§ 139. **Street cleaning.** The above described contrivances can also be used for the purpose of *street cleaning*, the object of which consists in removing as quickly as possible from the streets the dirt, the animal or vegetable refuse and the snow-masses. Impervious pavement of well-set plastering-stones, or blocks of wood or asphalt facilitates successful street-cleaning; for this reason this mode of paving is much used in recent times. Besides scavenging the streets, the labour of which is heaviest in winter and during wet weather, *regular sprinkling* (watering) of the streets is necessary during hot and dry weather to prevent the injurious dust, from being whirled up, as well as to cool the air (§ 38).

§ 140. **The supply of water.** A thorough cleansing of the soil removes many possible causes, which may lead to the *pollution of the water-courses* and wells; but this does not relieve from the duty of carefully surveying the springs and streams, which feed the supply of drinking and domestic water. Where *good* water is wanting or where the sources, whence the water is taken, are not protected from contamination, *the obtaining of pure, wholesome water* is one of the most urgent duties of the authorities, who are responsible for the hygiene. On this point it should be noted, that the *quantity* of the water supplied should correspond with the requirements of the population. It has been calculated, that the water supply then only corresponds to the wants of the people for drinking, washing and domestic purposes, as well as for street sprinkling, scavenging, and for gardening, fountains etc., if a daily supply of 150 litres for each inhabitant is allowed Where the capacity of the water works is not adequate for this, the *good* water ought not to be used for boilers, fountains and for watering the gardens, as these requirements can be satisfied by other water, drawn directly from river or ponds. It is also advisable, where the supply of good water is barely sufficient, to prevent waste of it by the people, either to limit the supply for each household to a certain quantity by the insertion of so-called "measuring cocks" into the pipes, or by "water-meters" in each dwelling; the latter contrivance ascertains the quantity of water, used in every household, and the population in thus induced to be sparing in their water consumption, as each surplus has to be paid for.

Where the efforts failed to obtain a supply of good water corresponding to the wants of the population, or where the standard of a daily supply of fifty litres for each inhabitant has not been reached, a *dearth of water* occurs. This entails consequences, injurious to health, as either the cleanliness in the household diminishes, or impure surface-water from rivers, ditches, ponds etc. is used for domestic purposes and as "drinking" water. If the water, supplied to the inhabitants of a place is purified by filtration, one is easily tempted during a water famine to allow the water to run too quickly through the filters; this permits larger quantities of water to be obtained; but the purity of it is diminished and under certain circumstances the health of the inhabitants is jeopardized.

§ 141. **The method of laying out a settlement.** In judging a settlement, its laying out plan must be taken into consideration in so far, as on it depends the ingress of light and air into each particular dwelling. In this connection the space of the settlement must be considered first; for fresh, wholesome air penetrates more easily into the narrow streets of a small town than into the wider streets in the heart of a great town. In places, which are surrounded by walls of a fortress the limited space necessitates the laying out of narrow streets and the building of high houses, while in an open town the construction of the houses can be made more in conformity with the requirements for light and air of the inhabitants.

The so-called "*Parzellen*" system, i. e. the system, which allows for *each* dwellighouse a site, open on all sides within a garden or courtyard presents the greatest advantages for health. This "lot" system however requires for its employment a large area in the settlement, which is inconvenient for traffic, and its use is rendered difficult in large towns by the high price of the real estate; one is therefore compelled to build dwelling-houses in towns in continuous *rows* and *groups*. The dwellings in these cases receive their fresh air and light mostly only from the streets and from the yards behind the houses; in the most favourable circumstances from open squares and gardens.

In towns great importance should be attached to the establishment of open *places* for *recreation*, adorned with flowers and trees; for they offer to many townspeople, especially the children a somewhat insufficient, but still necessary and welcome substitute for the open country. In modern times efforts are made to prevent a lack of fresh air and light in large towns by means of spacious courtyards and wide streets.

According to the building police regulations in Berlin the height of new buildings may not be more than 22 metres, and may not surpass the width of the courtyard by six metres; the new houses may not be built higher, than the street is wide.

The police regulations for buildings try to do the best for public hygiene; but these can only be applied for new buildings, and cannot be carried out in old towns or in the older districts of large cities. The streets in the new parts of towns are not always so arranged according to the prevailing directions of the wind and the position of the sun, as to make the access of light and air to each house as free as possible; the advantageous utilization of space, and the establishment of good communication between the central and the outlying parts of the town are still made the principal considerations in building towns or new settlements.

§ 142. **Dispersion of smoke, and other atmospheric impurities. The avoiding of nuisances from factories.** Special precautions should be taken to insure that the air will enter as pure as possible into the human dwellings in a town. Good arrangements for the removal of refuse promote the purity of the air, but alone are insufficient; for in the smoke, ascending from dwelling houses and factories as well as in the gases, diffused by the latter are to be found further sources of impurities in the atmosphere which, especially in towns injure the breathing of the inhabitants, who are obliged by their calling anyway to live far away from the open, pure, fresh air. Smoke and gases must be therefore thoroughly eliminated by suitable contrivances, or at least be carried by chimneys to such a height above the houses, that they will not pollute the lower atmospheric strata, intended for breathing. Manufactures, which cannot be carried on, even by the aid of careful arrangements and high chimneys without producing nuisances in their vicinity should be either established at a distance from human dwellings or be tolerated only on the outskirts of a large town. The same holds good for industries, which are impossible without loud noise, such as coppersmiths, circular saws, iron foundries and similar establishments. If the noise, caused by these works does not directly injure health, it destroys our comfort, and prevents the opening of windows, necessary for proper airing.

§ 143. Civilization and prosperity of the people. How far the demands of hygiene are attended to in the establishment and maintenance of a community depends on the *civilization* and *prosperity* of a people. The settlements of savage races are devoid of arrangements, indispensable for health, and a prosperous municipality more easily decides the construction of costly waterworks or the establishment of a regular transport of refuse, than a community, living in poor circumstances. — Moreover culture and wealth facilitate the pursuit of a healthy mode of life by the individual and thus contribute to strengthen his power of withstanding disease, while privations and improper conduct render the body of the starving and the uncivilized more exposed to injurious influences. The illness of the individual not only deprives the community of his labour, but also requires money for his nursing, and sometimes even exposes the other members of the community to the risk of contracting the disease.

An enlightened wealthy community readily grants to the town administration the right to make laws for the supervision of all institutions for the purpose of furthering the health of the community, and provides the pecuniary means for them.

§ 144. Provisions for the sale of food. Supervision of crowds, theatres, assembly rooms, pleasure resorts etc. The quality of the food of the people, is, as a rule left to the free rivalry of traders and industrial establishments; only in times of distress the public authorities take sometimes this care over, if need be to do so. Dishonesty and extortion are in this trade more reprehensible than in any other business, as it affects objects, which everyone, even the poorest has to buy every day, but of whose quality the purchaser is generally not in a position to judge. The public authorities have therefore the duty of instituting a strict supervision by experts of the trade in victuals and of suppressing the traffic in such victuals, which may be injurious to the health of the inhabitants from decomposition, adulteration or from other causes.

Such an injury can be found already in the misprensation of the quality of the food and the inducement to purchase it; for the buyer is thus led to spend money for a supposed necessary of life, and may have to retrench his purchases in real necessaries of life, which would be more conducive to health.

In Germany a law concerning *the sale of food* of May 14.th 1879 governs this important part of public hygiene. By this law police officers are empowered to enter shops, where articles of food are offered for sale and to take samples. The imitation or adulteration of food or refreshments with a view to deception of the trade; the sale of putrid, falsified, or adulterated food or refreshments, and the offering them for sale under a description, calculated to deceive purchasers is forbidden.

The *manufacture, sale or traffic in food* or refreshments or other articles of consumption, whose use is or may become injurious to health or may even destroy it, is forbidden by heavy penalties (prison, and even penal servitude).

As the application of these principles of public hygiene is not always easily feasible, and as the views of experts on these matters often differ, several special laws with regard to this matter were passed.

1. *Imperial law*, dated 24 February 1882, *concerning the sale of Petroleum*. Petroleom, which gives up imflammable vapour at a lower temperature than $21°$ C. may be sold only in vessels, bearing the inscription "inflammable" in large indelible characters in a prominent position.

2. *Law concerning the sale of objects, containing lead of zinc of* June 25 th 1887. Eating, drinking and cooking uteusils; then those portions of vessels and utensils employed in preserving fruit-juices which come in contact with the above mentioned food or refreshments may not be manufactured of lead or any alloy, containing more than ten percent of lead. They may not be coated inside with any metal, containing more than one percent of lead; they may not be soldered with any metal, that contains more than ten percent of lead; and may not be glazed or enameled inside with any matter, which after boiling with the ordinary vinegar ($4°/_0$) give off lead to the latter acid. Contrivances for the "draught" of beer, for siphons for mineral water or the metallic parts of infant's bottles may not be manufactured of metal, which contains more than one

percent of lead. Besides this law enumerates a large number of contrivances, toys and other objects in daily domestic use, which, if made of metal may not contain more than one percent of lead.

3. *A law concerning the use of colours, injurious to health in the manufacture of food, refreshments and other articles of domestic use*, of July 5th 1887. As colouring agents, injurious to health and therefore excluded from being used are mentioned the following: antimony, arsenic, barium, lead, cadmium, chromium, copper, mercury, uranium, zinc, tin, gamboge, corallin and picric acid. These colouring substances may not be used in wrappings, covers etc. for food or any other articles of domestic use, nor in articles for cleaning the skin; for making soap, in manufacturing toys, picture-books etc. Especially in printing — lithographing and similar work as well as in the manufacture of wall-paper, curtains, furniture-coverings and similar goods the use of colours containing arsenic is forbidden.

4. *Imperial ordnance*, dated February 1st 1891, *concerning the prohibition of machines for the production of artificial coffee-beans.*

5. *Law concerning the sale and trade in wine and winous drinks*, dated April 20th 1892, together with the carrying-out ordnance of this law, dated 29th April 1892. This law forbids the addition of a number of articles — injurious to health — to the above named beverages; furthermore forbids the sale of red wine, which contains more sulphuric acid, than the law permits. Certain processes for manufacturing wine are entirely prohibited, others only permitted under certain restrictions.

6. *Law concerning the trade in butter, cheese, lard etc.*, dated June 15th 1897. All shops, where vessels and utensils, in which and coverings of margarine butter and cheese and other artificial food of this class must bear in clear writing prominently on labels or otherwise the designation "margarine" or whatever name the artificial product bears. The mixing of genuine butter with margarine for trade purposes is not permitted. Margarine butter and cheese intended for trade must, to facilitate their chemical analysis contain 10 percent to 5 percent sesame oil respectively.

7. *Law concerning the trade in artificial sweetening stuffs*, dated July 6th 1898. This law forbids the employment of artificial sweetening stuffs for the preparation of beer, wine and similar beverages; fruit-juices, preserved fruit, liqueurs as well as of sugar and starch syrup. All other articles of food or refreshments, in the manufacture of which artificial sweetening stuffs are used, can only be sold, if such fact is made prominently known of a label.

A careful public authority is also in a position to ward off many dangers, which threaten the health of the people in their *public gatherings, amusements* etc. Accidents should be carefully guarded against at popular festivals, processions and similar displays by proper division of the crowds of people and at enclosed assemblies or public meetings by preventing the overcrowding of halls. The police authorities should also take care, that in assembly-halls, theatres, concert rooms and other pleasure resorts the construction of the halls as well as their ventilation, their heating and lighting contrivances should conform to the demands of public hygiene; furthermore that the "exits" for the public should be numerous and wide enough to allow these places to be emptied as quickly as possible; and that the public may disperse at all times, but particularly in case of fire quickly and without the danger of a crush.

§ 145. **Provision for the poor and sick.** To the duties of the government belongs also the *proper provision for the poor and sick*. By alleviating the necessities of the poor the development of epidemics is counteracted; because hunger and privations are the most favourable conditions for the development of general illnesses. The anxiety for their restoration to health must be lessened for the sick by the training of capable physicians, and of well-informed nurses, as well as by supervision of sick clubs and in the case of pauper sick by supplying proper food. The danger of improper treatment and of insufficient precautions against the communication of disease should be prevented by the restriction of quacks. Rules for the isolation of the sick, for disinfection and other rules should in certain cases prevent the further spread of infectious diseases.[1]) Purity of ingredients and scientific accuracy in compounding medicines is insured by a regulation of the status of *apothecaries*.

Persons, who desire to become apothecaries, must pass an examination. By various special laws certain compounds, the effect of which is violently strong, may not sold by the apothecaries without a doctor's prescription. The stock of medicines in every dispensary is examined occasionally by certain official doctors. The drug-book of the German Empire of 1901 is the standard book for judging the quality of the medicine. As *secret remedies* often substances recommended by quacks have obtained a large sale as means for the curing of many, especially tedious or incurable diseases. In many cases they are completely without value; frequently however they contain strongly acting substances, which should be used only after prescription by a doctor, and besides in most cases they are much dearer than they are worth. As their use frequently prevents people from calling in at the right time a genuine medical adviser, the public should be warned against the use of "secret medicines".

---

[1]) In Germany a law, dated June 30th 1900 was promulgated for combating infectious and contagious diseases; especially leprosy, cholera, typhus, yellow fever, plague and smallpox.

One essential means for promoting healthy conditions in human settlements is found in *infirmaries, hospitals* and *lunatic asylums*, which should be placed in an airy and healthy site, at some distance from the dwelling houses proper of the place and should be surrounded by gardens. In them the sick should receive medical aid, nursing, proper diet, medicines, bath and other remedies in such an irreproachable quality, that not only the poor, but also the wealthy people should find what is necessary for their recovery better executed in hospitals, than in their own dwellings; and the relatives of the patient, by being relieved of the duty of nursing the sick person, may be in a position to go about their business. These advantages, to which may be added the isolation of the sick in cases of epidemics are, however only fully realised in well-conducted hospitals; improperly conducted and badly arranged hospitals contribute to the spread of diseases by their liquid and solid refuse, and by the intercourse of those outside with the patients. With the civil authority therefore, in addition to the task of *erecting hospitals* lies the *duty* of *superintending* their internal arrangement and *management*.

§ 146. **Funerals.** In *burials*, as they are conducted generally in Germany the body is interred in a grave, about two metres deep, and then covered with earth. Putrefaction and decomposition then take place pretty quickly; in porous, sandy soil these processe ordinarily require from 4 to 7 years; but it takes a longer time in an unfavourable soil, such as loam or clay, before the fleshy parts of the human body are destroyed. The vitality of germs of disease, as far our knowledge goes is destroyed in a much quicker period of time; in any case these germs as well as the gases, produced by putrefaction and decomposition are kept from the surface of the earth by the layer of soil above the coffin. To avoid contamination of the ground water, places, where water is found only at a great depth should be selected as burial grounds.

Well arranged burial places are not dangerous to the health of the people in the neighbourhood, as neither tainting of the air, nor contamination of the water is caused by them. Children, who are carried by their nurses daily in the gardens, surrounding burial places thrive well, and very good spring water is found in wells near cemeteries. Only in those cases is the air not sufficiently protected from the gases arising in decomposition, and the surface of the earth is not safe from the germs of disease, where the graves are made too near the surface of the earth, i. e. not deep enough in the soil, or are covered with quick-sand, or where a burial ground is opened too soon after previous interments. Any peculiarity in the soil, which prevents decomposition, overcrowding, or the presence of water near the surface may lead to pollution of the water and the soil of the burial-ground. Such disadvantages cannot occur in well-managed burial-grounds; only in very exceptional cases they were observed; as for instance, when after battles or great accidents etc. a simultaneous interment of an unusually large number of corpses in a limited space has been found necessary; otherwise they may be wholly avoided.

The entombment of corpses in *vaults* is unobjectionable only, if the vaults are not overfilled, and especially, if the floor, walls and doors, locks etc. are absolutely tight and thick. These conditions are as a rule only fulfilled in the case of so-called "hereditary" vaults of single families; walled vaults, catacombs caves and similar places for entombment are not to be recommended for the purpose of general interment; for they do not insure the isolation of the corpses from living persons, and they must be frequently opened and visited.

Cremation, which in very recent time has been strongly recommended from various quarters, has not as yet been practised to any extent in Germany.

The fear of the possibility of burying still alive and only apparently dead persons is unfounded, if the regulations as to burial are rigidly carried out. The reports of cases of trance, which lasted longer, than the period prescribed by law between death and burial have proved on careful investigation to be untrue.

§ 147. Inspection of corpses. Disposal of corpses of persons, who have died of infectious diseases. By an inquest, or inspection of the corpse is meant ascertaining first the fact of death, and as far as possible also the cause of death, by means of an examination of the corpse by an expert, if possible by a physician; under special circumstances the body is opened to ascertain the cause of death. The ordering of this autopsy by law would insure many advantages, where it is possibly, and if properly carried out. It calms the relatives of the deceased, assists the administration of Law in detecting crimes, and promotes the observation of precautionary measures in regard to the corpses of persons, who have succumbed to infectious diseases.

The danger of communication of disease by corpses compels their speedy and trustworthy removal from the vicinity of living persons. It is therefore advisable to deposit corpses in isolated rooms or halls (*mortuaries*) in the cemetery until interment. Halls of this kind should be kept cool. In order to exclude as far as possible the danger of communicating disease during the transfer of the corpse to the mortuary or burial ground, the dead body is wrapped up in linen sheets, saturated with disinfecting fluids, prior to being exclosed in a perfectly tight coffin. Chance discharges from the corpse, prior to decomposition are absorbed by sawdust, turf mould etc. spread at the bottom of the coffin and are thus prevented from becoming visible. The destruction of particularly dangerous disease germs, which might be present in the body may occasionally require quicklime to be scattered in the coffin and in the grave.

§ 148. **Removal of dead animals.** Similar considerations in regard to health, as are taken into account in the burial of dead persons, also determine the removal of dead animals. As a rule the carcases of large animals are buried in remote spots which fulfil the same conditions, as are necessary for human burial-grounds. Dead animals are more quickly destroyed by burning, or by being used up in the manufacture of glue, manure etc. The persons who follow the business of removing animal carcases are called *knackers* or *skinners*.

There are special laws for the removal of dead animals, which died in consequence of "Rinderpest", anthrax, glanders, or rabies. These laws are dated 23 June 1880 and May 1st 1894.

II. Commerce.

§ 149. **Objects of commerce. Means of communication.**

The manifold relations and points of contact, which exist among men in their settlements are increased by traffic from place to place, from country to country. Commercial intercourse between individuals and nations has existed since the most ancient times of which we have historic knowledge. Travelling was however up to a few decades ago so difficult or costly, that the number of persons, who resolved to leave their homes and undertake distant journeys, whether for pleasure or instruction, for industrial or commercial purposes or on account of their profession was very small. Where not willing to reach their destination by troublesome walking, considerable sums had to be spent for horses and carriages, and even when journeying by water was available, the ship's voyage was of uncertain duration, because it depended upon the direction and strength of the wind.

Since then the means of transit have been perfected in an unexpected manner by the ever-increasing application of steam, and recently of electricity. To-day a distant journey entails little trouble, time and money, compared with former years, and the number of persons travelling every year and the quantity of goods conveyed has increased enormously, so that according to the Imperial word „the present time stands under the signature of commerce".

§ 150. Travelling. The expansion of traffic has caused certain consequences on human health to appear more prominently or differently than before. For the individual travelling at present appears to be not only more comfortable, but also more healthy than formerly. Legal regulations and government inspections prevent uncleanliness and overcrowding in carriages and provide for their necessary ventilation, heating and lighting. The arrangements for the health and comfort of travellers on railways and steamboats are being constantly improved and it frequently happens nowadays, that persons seriously ill can be conveyed to far-distant places without incurring any risk by travelling.

The impression conveyed from the number of railway and steamboat accidents, that the danger of travelling has increased by reason of the modern means of conveyance must be declared as erroneous. The accidents are extraordinarily small in number as compared with the immense increase of traffic. They appear terrible to many only because, as a rule, a greater number of persons are implicated at the same moment in an accident than before, and because the newspapers spread the news of an accident more quickly; whereas formerly accidents were almost always limited in the number of victims in accordance with the mode of conveyance, and easily escaped the notice of the public.

Injuries to health by travelling can rarely be laid to the door of the condition of the vehicles for conveyance; but an individual traveller may fall ill on a journey through his own imprudent or careless conduct. Travelling makes various and many demands on the body; our customary way of living is altered; for in place of the accustomed food we obtain another diet, we have to eat at different hours, and sleep must be sought at different hours from our usual time of going to bed. Besides, the quick change of climate occasioned by travelling from one place to another may endanger the health; and no small risk arises from the possibility of catching disease through contact with strangers and by spending the night in strange rooms and beds. When travelling we should be even more moderate in our mode of life than ordinarily, we should avoid excesses of every kind, which might reduce our power of resistance and endurance and we should protect ourselves by proper clothing from sudden changes of temperature and other meteorological influences. In railway carriages we should provide pure air by suitable use of the ventilating apparatus and by judicious opening of the window; but we should avoid causing injurious draughts of air and should not lean out of the window. Many a man has lost his life owing to such imprudent conduct, when a door of the compartment flew open in consequence of the weight of his body, and many eyes have been injured by the keen draft or by dust or cinders, when the traveller put his head out of the window. Moreover one should lodge and board only in clean, conscientiously conducted hotels, and we should avoid too close contact with strangers. During long journeys we should occasionally take a day's rest to protect the body from over-exertion.

§ 151. **Prevention of the spread of infectious diseases by traffic.** If the perfecting of the modes of conveyance has been rather an advantage for the travelling individual, it has on the other hand increased the danger of spreading infectious diseases for the general public. The increase of traffic, and the speed, with which at present long distances are traversed by land and by sea favours the possibility of introducing contagious diseases and hastens their progress from place to place.

Various efforts have been made to meet this danger of introducing illnesses. Either the frontiers of the countries were closed, or the local boundaries of such places, where contagious diseases prevailed were shut against all traffic from such dangerous localities; or persons coming from there had to spend a certain time in quarantine — up to forty days — and submit to an examination with reference to their health, and to have all their luggage disinfected, before they were permitted to cross the frontier; finally the importation of all goods, from which an importation of the disease is feared, was forbidden or allowed only after disinfection. As a rule, the end in view was not obtained by all these regulations, in spite of all the highly inconvenient molestations, which were seriously felt by travellers and by commerce.

§ 152. **Closure of frontiers; Quarantines.** The complete suspension of traffic from outside the frontier may be possible in small remote places or on islands; in all other cases however, especially on a *land frontier* it is regularly broken, as experience teaches; in spite of large numbers of guards, specially sent for watching the frontier. In many cases even the guards were the persons who caught the infection from the travellers and spread the disease.

Of course it is easier to prevent vessels coming oversea from getting into the harbour, or to prevent intercourse with the shore within the limits of the port, until the time of observation has elapsed. But even the result of these *sea quarantines* has not corresponded to expectations; as cases of sickness, which occurred on board during the time of observation were concealed or remained undetected, and have subsequently become the source of further cases of the disease in the port. Much more effective for the prevention of epidemies seems a constant medical supervision of the state of health in the ports.

The regulations, directed against the import of inanimate objects were often too stringent. Cases are known, of course, where the contagious disease was actually transmitted by packages, postal parcels etc.; but the number of such cases is very small indeed, and there are only a few objects, which with some degree of certainty can be accused of spreading a contagious disease. — But even rags, feathers, wool etc., whose capacity of absorbing and spreading the germs of many infectious diseases is undisputable, may be safely forwarded, when carefully packed and securely closed; if their further use at their destination is permitted only after disinfection under very stringent supervision.

§ 153. **Measures against the spreading of epidemics in Germany.** Experience during the last cholera epidemics in Germany taught, that general epidemics can be combated effectively without troublesome measures blocade. To prevent the introduction of *cholera* into districts, which are not yet "infected" persons, coming from "cholera infected" places are subjected to observation during several days without however essentially interfering with free traffic. Isolation takes place in cases of illness only. Stricter supervision, in certain circumstances even restrictions of traffic only take place against persons without fixed domicile, vagrants, people without a permanent home or place of abode; against gypsies, tramps, foreign vagabonds, and the occupants of river boats or rafts. Besides, popular festivals (Volksfeste), fairs, pilgrimages etc. are prohibited immediately threatened with the epidemic; because the disease was often spread far and wide — as experience showed — by the crowds, coming together on such occasions. The experience, gathered during the cholera epidemic is also valuable for combating other epidemics, especially the epidemic of the plague. Restrictions of goods traffic are only ordered under certain conditions in regard to milk, old and worn clothes, old bedding, rags etc.

§ 154. **Other risks through goods traffic.** Danger to health is not restricted to the possibility of introducing an epidemic disease, so far as goods traffic is concerned. The conveyance of food, refreshments, and other provisions for great distances sometimes causes these goods to become putrid on the journey, and thus produces sickness among the receivers or purchasers. In packing these objects and stowing them away on railways, boats etc. the precautionary measures, mentioned in § 86 and 100 must be especially observed. It is also advisable to consume food sent from abroad only, when we have assured ourselves that no signs of decomposition can be perceived on them.

III. Education.

§ 155. General influence of education. A considerable progress, attained by the union of men into communities lies in the increased mental culture of the people. The emulation of the nations in securing and improving their circumstances compels them to set the aims of popular culture higher than formerly and to provide, that a certain minimum of knowledge be acquired by every healthy child. Primary school education becomes therefore a vital question to every civilized nation. While formerly it was left to the individual citizen in which manner he wanted to bring up and to educate his children, their *compulsory attendance* in a school is now enforced by law. This however extends only to the attendance in the primary school, i. e. to instruction in knowledge which is absolutely necessary in our daily life. Some professions however require a more extensive general education in a preparatory school as a necessary basis for the understanding of our duties and for the success of our future work in life. For these requirements is adapted a course of education, extending over a longer period at the higher technical schools and universities. By a *onesided* cultivation of the intellect the bodily powers are hindered in their development and lowered; not only the individual suffers through a general neglect of physical development, but the entire people also is a sufferer; the decline in bodily strength increases from one generation to the next, and the enfeebled nation is no longer able to make a stand against the foreign enemy. It is therefore the duty of parents and teachers as well as of the state to watch that the rising population should be well cared for and protected from injurious influences and that the necessary training of the intellect should not interfere with the healthy development of the juvenile body.

§ 156. Mortality of infants. At no other period is man's life in such danger as in his earliest infancy. During 1898, according to the reports of the Imperial Board of Health $36._5$ per cent of the deaths in the German Empire, 40 per cent of those in Bavaria, $36._6$ per cent of the deaths in Berlin were infants under one year of age; in other countries and towns death also claimed numerous victims among children of that tender age. Of every 100 children born alive in Germany during 1898 died in the German Empire 20.8 per cent, (cf. above), in Prussia 19.3 per cent, in Bavaria 25.9 per cent and in Saxony 25.4 per cent during the first year of their life, so that at that time in the above mentioned states only ¾ of all children born alive survived the first year of their life. The extent of infant mortality is subject to considerable fluctuations according to the time of the year and to the locality. About a third of all the cases of death among children of this tender age occurs during the months of July and August, and in the large towns the mortality among infants is usually considerably higher, than among a rural population. Particularly many more children, born out of wedlock die during the first year of their life than legitimate children, evidently because they obtain less care and nursing than children, who are brought up by their legitimate parents.

§ 157. **The food for infants.** The most frequent illnesses of the first year of the life of an infant are caused by improper nourishment. Many mothers cannot, others will not suckle their babies, whether from reasons of health or of their occupation, or as it unfortunately often happens, without any reason that could be morally justified. Only a few wealthy parents can afford to provide a somewhat complete substitute by hiring a wet-nurse; the greater majority of those children have to do without their natural nutriment — mother's milk. In such cases milk of the cow or other animals forms their chief nourishment; this is indeed the most suitable substitute next to mother's milk; but it should be obtained as pure as possible, kept free from impurities and well boiled before being used (cf. §§ 75—77). Stupid mothers, who want to provide for their children during the first months of their life too strong (rich) nourishment in the shape of pure or little thinned milk, often cause the child's stomach, injured by the heavy diet either partially to reject the food, or they induce, serious disorders of the digestive organs.

Many children thrive also, if they receive milk substitutes (§ 77), along with animal (fresh) milk. Well-boiled and thoroughly-strained soups, made from oats, barley or other cereals may also be given to children more than three months old as an additional food to their milk; but one ought not to forget that the nutritive quality of such soups is far less than that of milk. A too premature attempt to nourish a child with the food of an adult person is almost always punished by severe digestive disorders.

The dreaded dysenteries of the infantile period are frequently the consequences of neglect of cleanliness in keeping and handling the milk supply; hence they cause more cases of death among children, fed on animal milk or farinaceous substitutes for mother's milk, among children, fed at their mother's breast.

Light baked bread (biscuits, cakes) can be eaten by infants without injury ordinarily not before the last three months of the first year of their life; soft boiled eggs and easily digestible meat (§ 82) after the first year. Children ought not to get light vegetables, potatoes and fruit before the expiration of the first year of their life. Subsequently children easily get accustomed to a stronger diet; but food difficult to digest or strongly spiced dishes and spirituous liquors ought to be entirely withheld from them. Pampering with sweetstuffs and other delicacies is a bad habit which not only injures their education but also undermines the health of children by leading to diseases of the teeth and other digestive disorders (cf. § 58).

§ 158. **Baths. Children's clothing. Necessity of fresh air. Eye-diseases of newly-born infants. Sleep. Causes of children's crying.** Cleanliness is an indispensable requirement of the proper bringing up of children. For the thriving of children it is necessary that they should be bathed every day, that their hair and the folds in the skin should be carefully cleaned and that those parts of the body, most exposed to dirt should be powdered and in certain cases also greased. The skin of children, to whom such proper treatment is not given easily becomes sore and covered with eruptions which hinder the development of the child's body.

The infant body is very sensitive to *chills*; hence for the bath warm water of about 34^0 C. ($27-28^0$ R.) should be taken, and the children ought to be provided with warm clothing and bedding. It is a very stupid fear however to deprive them of fresh air out in the open. If the fear of catching cold and wettings is not grounded by a strong high wind or by rain or snow, healthy infants should be taken into the open air already daily a few weeks after birth.

Special attention should be paid to *the eyes of newly-born babies.* The dreaded disease of the eye (cf. § 219) which without proper professional care usually leads to blindness of the infants can always be cured by prompt treatment. There should be no delay in sending for the Doctor as soon as red eyes, closed eye-lids or drops of mucous in the corners of the eyes show the beginning of an inflammation. Daylight is not injurious to the eye of a healthy child, unless the sun shines too glaringly through the windows.

Quiet must prevail in the nursery, as the newly-born baby in the first months of its life requires a good deal of sleep.

The *crying* of babies often represents only the expression of awakened life; it is the language in which the infant makes known its wants. A child cries sometimes, because it is hungry, and becomes quieter, as soon as the quantity of food is increased or its composition altered. The cause of its crying may be sometimes a wet „diaper" or the pressure of some improperly arrangend article of clothing. The fear that illness is the cause of baby's crying is seldom well founded; on the contrary; a strong voice is not without reason considered as a sign of health.

§ 159. Cutting the teeth. Development of speech. Standing and walking. The *cutting of the teeth*, usually beginning during the second six months of life causes much discomfort. Painful swelling of the gums sets in, saliva is largely secreted; the children often put their fingers into their mouths, sleep uneasily and are generally tearful and fretful. Slight feverishness may also be traced to the teeth. Other symptoms of illness frequent at this period of life, such as eruptions, spasmodic convulsions, coughs, high fever etc. have usually nothing to do with cutting the teeth and are at most made worse by their simultaneous appearance. The custom of ascribing all illness at this time of life to the cutting of the teeth and for this reason omitting to call in a physician sometimes brings in its own punishment in the death of the child.

Towards the end of the first year the child begins to babble the first words. The *development of speech* is accomplished as a rule without difficulties and is not influenced by the nature of the cord which joins the tongue to the bottom of the oral cavity. If the cord is too short or somewhat tight, it is gradually extended by the movements in speech.

III. Education. 153

The loosening of the tongue by a slit in the cord is superfluous, and may give rise to inflammation as well as to festering. At the same age children begin to stand and to walk. They require then careful supervision, lest they may injure themselves by falling. In many cases, as a consequence of weakness of the bones caused by a disease, called "rickets" *(rachitis)* or so-called English malady the inclination to learn to walk is shown rather later. To encourage such children to walk is imprudent; long lying is advantageous for them, as their limbs become deformed in walking owing to the weight of their body.

§ 160. **Awakening of intellect; Kindergarten.** Gradually the awakening of the faculty of thinking, the dawning of intelligence, and the development of a will-power demand for the child the *education of his mind* in addition to the care for his body. The more respect that is paid to natural development in this direction and the less the infant faculty of comprehension is burdened with ideas of which he stands in no need yet, the healthier develops his understanding, his mind. To parents, who from their profession, illness, or other impediments are prevented from devoting their own time and labour to the education of their children, the *kindergarten* offer welcome assistance. There the children enjoy themselves in common games and at the same time receive the first useful instruction. The conditions of space and fittings of kindergärten are to be regulated by the same rules, as the schools so far as hygiene is concerned.

§ 161. **School hours; duties of the government, the masters, physicians-teachers and parents.** With his entry into the schoolroom a notable change takes place in the mode of life of the child. A part of the day is spent in a prescribed occupation; mental as well as bodily exertions are demanded and the child learns what is meant by *"duty"*.

The sense of justice demands, that in a state, where attendance at school is compulsory, the children should be exposed as little as possible to dangers to health, while in school. It is the duty of the headmaster of the school to see to it, according to the standard laid down by the regulations of the state for schools, that neither the arrangements in the class-rooms, nor the mode of instruction does any injury to the health of the children; the teachers should observe each individual pupil, and pay attention to the peculiarities — cf the body as well as of the mind — of each child. In a great many German schools, special school physicians have been engaged, whose duty it is to examine carefully at stated periods the schoolrooms and their fittings, to urge the amelioration of existing faulty arrangements, and in general to watch constantly over the health of the school-children and to order, if necessary such measures conducting to improvement of the health of the pupils.

This however does not exempt the parents and tutors at home from their duties towards their children. The observation of the child's conduct during leisure hours, of his appetite and sleep leads much more easily than is possible during school hours to the discovery of derangements of health or defects in his development. Often an explanation with a teacher or head of the school leads to timely discovery and prevention of danger threatening the child's health. Suitable treatment at home, bodily exercise, walks, proper management of irregularities strengthen the power and capacity for undergoing the efforts, required by school instruction.

§ 162. **The schoolhouse and the schoolroom.** The *requirements of a schoolhouse* are in the first place those of a dwelling-house (cf. § 111—131), but the class-rooms proper must fulfil besides special conditions. Their length, width, and height should not exceed a certain standard, because the writing on the black board must be capable of being read from the hindmost form without special effort; the seats near the wall furthest from the window must receive sufficient light and the sound must not be injured by too high a ceiling. As a rule these conditions are fulfilled by a schoolroom not more than ten metres long, seven metres wide and about four metres high; and such a room, having an air capacity of nearly 280 cubic metres would accomodate about fifty children in the lowest standard. If the space reserved for each child is small (cf. § 116) it must be borne in mind, that schoolrooms are occupied continuously only for a short time. But, so large an attendance is only permissible on condition, that in the intervals between lessons a thorough renewal of the air in the room is insured by opening the doors and windows, and that suitable contrivances provide constant ventilation during the hours of study.

The choice of heating apparatus for a school-house is determined usually by the climate and other local conditions, as well as by the size of the building. For large schools a collective heating system combined with ventilating apparatus is generally preferred. Experience proves a schoolroom temperature of $18°$ C. to be sufficient for the pupils.

The walls, floors and fittings of a schoolroom should be as level as possible; nowhere should corners, joinings or crevices afford resting places for dirt or dust. An accumulation of dangerous refuse (§ 49) can be prevented only by regular (several times a week) scouring and washing up of the floors etc.

A vice, frequently developed already in early childhood is spitting; children should be restrained from acquiring this evil habit on grounds of good breeding and cleanliness, and only in cases of illness should children be permitted to expectorate. Such coughing pupils however should be strictly enjoined to expectorate into "spittoons" and not on the floor — in the schoolroom as well as out of school. — Expectorating on the floor might result in disease-germs becoming mixed with the dust of the room, the breathing of which might become injurious to the other children.

§ 163. Relation between the lighting of the schoolroom and the origin of short-sight. The lighting of the schoolroom is very important in regard to health; for defective light helps to produce short-sightedness and curvature of the spine, to which children are subjected. A sickly bodily disposition frequently lies at the root of both defects; the development of short sight is however favoured by the exertions, required from the eyes, when reading, writing or drawing in badly lighted rooms, just as spinal curvature easily appears in young persons, if they have to bend their head constantly near the table in the effort to place their eyes close to the badly lighted paper or book. The daylight must not be prevented by trees, houses or walls from penetrating into the schoolroom; from every seat in all forms a part of the sky ought to be seen. High, wide windows (according to the Wurtemberg school-law of about $\frac{1}{5}$ the floor-space) ought to afford free, plentiful access to the daylight; light gray or bluish tinted walls, to be kept free from dust, favour the diffusion of light and do not dazzle the eyes. It is best for the light to fall in from the left or from above the pupil's seat; if it comes from the front, it dazzles; if from the back, the child's shadow obscures the surface of the desk before him; if the light comes from the right, the pupils are disturbed by the shadow of their hand or their pen, and are thus induced to sit crooked. If daylight on dull winter's days proves insufficient, artificial lighting should be plentiful (cf. § 125, 127). The books and copies, used by pupils during lessons should not exert the eyes by too small print or faded lines. Maps are best made without too "loud" colours, and should not, as is prescribed by the Wurtemberg school-law represent too much simultaneously; i. e. they should not try to show on the same map geographical and political divisions of the earth, together with the rivers, or mountain ranges etc., all gaily illuminated.

§ 164. **School-forms; curvatures of the spine.** The formation of the school bench and desk has great importance upon either favouring or preventing spinal curvature. Negligence in main-

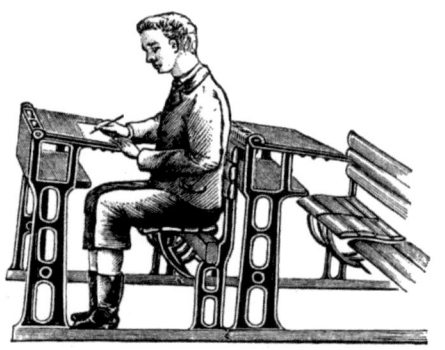

Fig. 40.
Pupil writing in good position.

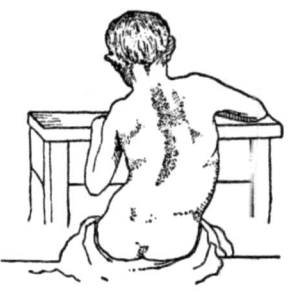

Fig. 41.
Writing pupil in defective position
(after v. Esmarch).

taining the upright position of the body is most easily avoided, if the pupil can assume and maintain the upright position without muscular effort (Fig. 40). A high seat, which, when the knees are bent at right angles does not allow the feet to rest on the floor, or a narrow bench, which does not afford room for the whole upper thigh, tires the muscles of the legs. If the lid of the desk is too low, and not high enough from the bench, the pupil is compelled to an inconvenient stooping of his head. If the desk is too high, it makes it difficult to place the right arm on it and causes an elevation of the right shoulder; and at the same time the eye must be brought injuriously near to the desk (Fig. 41). Too great a distance between the back of the desk and the front of the seat causes necessarily a bending of the spine "strains the muscles of the back and hinders respiration. In order to guard against the pupil's deportment relaxing by weariness of the muscles of the back, or against formation of permanent curvature of the vertebral column, the benches are to be manufactured in such a manner, that with a slight bend in the seat of the bench the pupil in his sitting postition should have a strengthening of the bending of the vertebral column.

In recent years the school authorities are endeavouring to adapt the lighting arrangements of the schoolroom and the school benches to hygienic requirements. Still there are children, who fail to sit upright even in well-lit rooms and on proper seats. It is then generally a question of a bad habit, which the pupil should be urged to lay aside; in exceptional cases the faulty carriage may be due to illness, which may take a disastrous course unless timely treatment is sought; therefore parents and teachers should occasionally ask medical advice. Some physicians recommend the introduction of the "steep" writing style for the pourpose of obtaining an upright position of the pupils.

The injurious effect of sitting crooked is displayed not merely in short-sightedness and spinal curvature; it sometimes occasions interruptions in the circulation of the blood; so that it may lead to effusion of blood in the brain, headache and bleeding from the nose.

§ 165. **The alleged over pressure of pupils. Injudicious division of school-lessons.** Some persons in recent time have ascribed the above named injuries to health of the pupils to over-exertion and have thereupon accused the higher schools of overtasking the children, entrusted to them. This reproach however is as a rule not justifiable and frequently exaggerated. A certain amount of exertion must be asked from the pupil, as not only the teaching of the youths is the duty of the public schools, but also their training to become industrious an dutiful citizens. Among other things home exercises are indispensable, as the pupil then only learns to think for himself, when he is compelled to work alone. The plan of studies in the German public schools is throughout adapted to the working capacity of children and youths and careful supervision by the state and the school boards insures that no teacher should overtax the working capacity of his pupils. If however in spite of these precautions some pupils show signs of over-exertion in being discontented or easily excited, or being stunted in their physical development, or by falling ill, then in most cases other circumstances are to blame, most frequently an improper division of work. If the preparation of home work is only begun a short time before it has to be handed in to the teacher, and the hours, not occupied by instruction are exclusively devoted to play and pleasure, then the night time must be devoted to home exercises, and the period of sleep, with which children and youths cannot dispense without injury to their health, is shortened, and the pupils are not able during day-time to follow their lessons in school with the necessary freshness and attention. At the same time the home exercises, which in such cases are plainly performed with a certain reluctance, do not meet with the teacher's approval; the memory and understanding of the pupil do not sufficiently assimilate the material, supplied to them, and then the pupil's efforts must in fact be increased beyond his capacity, if the desired gaol of advancing into a higher class and a satisfactory final-certificate is to be attained.

§ 166. **Mode of life during the period of life, when the child is compelled to school-attendance.** The evils, just described become still more prominent by an injudicious mode of life. A proper care of the body should go hand in hand with the development of the mind. The recreation hours, and especially the holidays should be devoted to walks, gymnastics, swimming, skating etc. and not spent indoors. The diet of a growing youth should be simple; early habits of alcoholic drinks and tobacco undermine the health, and should be carefully avoided. Staying up late at night has injurious effects and therefore bringing schoolboys to the amusements of adults, whereby often late hours are taken up, is very injudicious. To the growing boy or girl the participation in all noisy assemblies, the holding of fashionable children's "parties", the visiting of theatres and concerts should not be permitted, or only in quite exceptional cases; for all such pleasures have generally the result, that they withdraw the pupil's thoughts from serious lessons and their duties. The same holds good of improper books; such as histories of revolting crimes, and many novels, whose perusal excites the mind of undeveloped persons excessively. It has happened, that by reading bad books the ideas of morality and honour have become so distorted, that pupils of an unbalanced mind have not shrunk from suicide from extraordinary motives. On the other hand supplying good books, which awake a sense of right and the appreciation of beautiful forms and thoughts is both advisable and beneficial, and those recreation hours should be given to them, which unfavourable weather does not permit to be spent in the open air. Instruction in music and the other arts is recommended exclusively for boys and girls who have a taste in that direction; and even in their case care must be taken, that their additional work does not interfere with their school work, nor shorten their hours of recreation, so as to avoid over-exertion.

§ 167. Development and protection of the body in the schools. Gymnastic training. The physical development of boys and girls should not be overlooked in schools. The teachers should observe the deportment of their pupils, give them proper advice and admonish them, and draw the attention of their parents to it either by remarks in the certificates or by personal observations in good time, where home interference is necessary. Pupils, suffering from contagious diseases should be kept apart from the others, or be exempted from school attendance along with their brothers and sisters, until the danger of infection ist past; in more extensive outbreaks of infectious diseases the classes or schools affected should be entirely closed for a time (school physicians § 161). Gymnastic training promotes the strength and the agility of the body and its members; attention should be paid to defects of a child. But anxious parents act injudiciously, if they prevent their children without sufficient cause to take part in gymnastic training and useful bodily exercise. The injuries occasionally sustained in gymnastic exercise are almost always of a trivial character, and give no occasion for its prohibition, since such accidents would be perhaps more frequent without gymnastic training. Boys require tumbling about and would perhaps seek to satisfy their craving for it in more violent games without supervision, that if gymnastics fell into disuse.

§ 168. Capacity of pupils. If children, in spite of their obvious efforts are unable to master the tasks, set them in school, and give rise to the fear, that their health may be injured by overstudy, the question presents itself to parents and teachers, whether the selected mode of instruction is not disproportioned to the pupil's capacity. Sometimes a change of school may still be useful, if one can select instead of a large school a smaller one, where the teacher can devote himself more to each individual pupil; but if this mode of changing matters is of no avail, and if laziness or negligence can with certainty be excluded as the cause of the lack of progress, no further time should be lost to change the mode of instruction. Many a pupil, who finds insuperable difficulties in learning languages understands the problems of Euclide quite easily; and physical skil or power of sharp observation secure a high position in life to many a man, who would only play a very subordinate role in a scientific profession.

The decision with regard to a change in the class of instruction is made easier to the parents by consulting with the teacher and the physician; the child's wish should not always be conclusive; for youth very easily errs in its wishes; and the craving, whose fulfilment closes many a profession frequently repented, when the understanding has become more natured.

§ 169. Girl's education in particular. Special care must be taken in the education of girls; for they require much more attention and observation than boys; over-exertion of their tender bodies often revenges itself in chlorosis (anæmia) irritability, nervosity and other indispositions. Girl's schools should therefore avoid all over-pressure of the pupils entrusted to them, and mothers should lovingly guard and teach their daughters. Only girls, whose mental capacities and healthy physical state guarantees their fitness should be selected for the training for the labourious professional and other work, which society has now opened to women also.

IV. Profession and business.

§ 170. Advantages and disadvantages of special occupations in relation to health. Factory inspectors. As soon as the school-years are over, training for their future occupation begins with most young men. Many even during this period of training, but all at the end of their apprenticeship are subject to new influences, determined by the class of occupation which they chose. Whether it is a question of factory-workers, handicrafts-men, agricultural labourers, artists, officials or savants, the individual is generally placed in the *peculiar relations* of his calling, which may exert a favourable or unfavourable influence on his health.

Scientific inquiry has been lately particularly directed to the discovery of the injurious results of various trades on the persons engaged in them. Inquiries in that respect have been ordered by the state, as the pursuit of a number of trades was placed under the supervision of special officials, — *factory inspectors* — who besides discharging other funtions are entrusted with the duty of reporting as to the healthy or unhealthy character of certain trades. The knowledge acquired in this way, which is continually being enlarged, has in many cases already made it possible to counteract injurious influences, either by perfecting the arrangements for the well-being of the workers, or by special laws, or Government regulations.

A complete removal of dangers in workshops is impossible, the object of the efforts, referred to must be rather be to confine the risks of every trade within the smallest possible limits, compatible with the purpose, for which the working is designed. Too far-reaching precaution or supervision would result in this: that with the removal of the danger a decrease of the labour would follow, and that the individual as well as the persons combined for the purpose of common work, and finally the whole nation could no longer exist in competition with other less considerate workers and nations.

§ 171. Importance of choice of profession — Prevention of weakly persons from entering in labourious occupations. Limitation of hours of labour for women and childern. The suitable choice of occupation is essentially important. He who devotes himself to an occupation without the physical capacity necessary for it generally suffers most easily from its injurious effects. Therefore; the admission to many industrial occupations, for instance mining, or the employment cn railways, or the service in the army and navy is made dependent on a *satisfactory bodily examination*. Previous to entering into a profession, which demands particularly brainwork, the *mental capacity* for it should be examined of course. The applicants should produce evidence for their aptitude for the work and of the degree of maturity of their mind. The employment of women and children in trades, which demand heavy bodily work is by law either restricted or forbidden.

According to the law concerning industrial occupations of June 1. 1891 for the German Empire children under 13 years of age may not be employed at all in factories; children over 13 only in the case, when their attendance in school is no longer obligatory. Besides, the Federal Council has the right to forbid the employment of women workers or juvenile workers in certain trades, which are either especially dangerous to health or to morality. In pursuance of this, the Federal Council has fixed by a great number of special law the trades and industries, where and at what age young girls and boys may not be employed, or only for a few hours daily, or only after they have reached the 16th year. Women after their accouchement cannot be employed at all in factories until four weeks have elapsed, and during the two weeks after the first month only on a certificate of health by an official physician.

In pursuance of an Imperial order of 31 May 1897 the regulations of the Trade ordinance concerning the work of women, children and juvenile workers should also be of legal force in the work-shops of the clothes and cloths manufactures ("Wäsche-Confeotion").

As the state however can influence the choice of calling only to a limited extent without encroaching on personal freedom, the responsibility for chosing a trade after a conscientious estimate of capacity as compared with the labour entailed rests chiefly with the individual, his parents or guardians.

§ 172. Duration of daily work. In every occupation too prolonged *duration of daily work* in proportion to man's working power may prove injurious to health; still it is difficult to lay down a standard time, which may be uninterruptedly devoted to work without entailing injury to the worker (§ 132). Not only must the class of business be taken into account, but also the personal working capacity and the way, in which the individual works. Some work slowly; some quickly; one man requires many short intervals of rest, another is refreshed by less frequent, but more extended interruptions of his work. A uniform determination of the

IV. Profession and business.

working time is unavoidable in industries, requiring the employment of many persons in the same way. In the German Empire the hours of work for each factory are regulated by *special regulations* of the *ordinance for labour* (a special law for factories). Moreover the Federal Council has the right of prescribing the duration, beginning and ending of admissible daily work and the obligatory intervals during working hours for factories, in which excessive length of daily work may be injurious to the health of the workman.

The Federal Council has promulgated laws with reference to bakers and pastry-cooks, electrical and accumulator works, mills and all industries, where lead combinations are worked. In open retail shops the shop must be closed between 9 in the evening and 5 in the morning. Under certain conditions the closure can be ordered by the Government at 8 and the opening not before 6 or 7 o'clock in the morning. In shops and offices the employes (clerks etc.) must obtain after working hours ten hours of uninterrupted rest; in towns with more than 20.000 inhabitants and shops or offices with more than 2 employes these must obtain at least 11 hours rest; besides an suitable time of rest at noon, which cannot be less than 1½ hours for all employes, who have to take their meals out of the house where the shop or office is situated.

The length of the working day for the juvenile and for the female worker is fixed by law.

According to the industrial law childern under 14 years of age cannot be employed in factories for more than 6 hours daily, juveniles between 14 and 16 not more than 10 hours daily. Female workers even over 16 years of age must not be kept at work for more than 11 hours daily, on the saturday and days before holidays not more than 10 hours; and in general not after 5¼ o'cl. in the afternoon, for meals at noon they must have at least one hour rest, and if they have a household of their own 1½ hours rest for the midday rest.

An important step in recognizing man's need of recreation by legal enactments has taken place by the introduction of the regulations concerning the *Sunday rest*, to which considerations for religion as well as considerations of health have given occasion.

According to the *industrial law* workmen as a rule cannot be asked to work on sundays and holidays. The work in mines, building places, salt-mines, wharfs, brickmaking and such-like work must be stopped altogether on sundays and holidays; only in exceptional cases or where delay might cause unavoidable damage the Federal Council may grant special permissions. Apart from these special laws the period of rest on Sundays should be at least 24 hours, for two successive holidays at least 36 hours, for Christmas, Easter and the Whit-holidays 48 hours; the period of rest commences at midnights and lasts until six o'cl. P. M. on the following day. Industries with regular day and night shifts the rest must commence at the earliest at 6 P. M. the day before or the latest at 6 o'cl. A. M. on the day of the holiday. In shops or trades or offices apprentices, clerks, workmen etc. may not be employed at all on the first day of Christmas, Easter and Whitholidays; on Sundays and other holidays not more than during 5 hours. By municipal regulations these hours for working may be either shortened or extended. Juvenile workers must not be employed at all during Sunday and holidays.

§ 173. **Injuries to health by overworking certain parts of the body.** In addition to general over-exertion due to a difficult or prolongued labour beyond our strength the *special exertion of certain parts of our body*, such as certain groups of muscles or sense organs may have injurious results. Persons, who write or sew much, play the piano or engage in other occupations, demanding constant exercise of the muscles of the hand and forearm, sometimes contract a troublesome disease of the nerves, best known as *writer's cramp*. The occupation of savants, watchmakers, goldworkers etc. necessitating much work with small objects with manuscripts or print injure the *power of vision*. Glaring light combined with sudden changes between brightness and darkness and radiated heat frequently produce illnesses of the eyes in the case of blacksmiths and glass-workers.

The constant posture, required by callings, which interferes with the circulation of the blood and other functions of the body, may cause injurious effects. The bent position of the upper part of the body, required by the work of shoemakers, tailors and sempstresses restricts the expansion of the chest and in this way sometimes leads to asthma, tic and pulmonary diseases. Long sitting obstructs the circulation of the blood and the intestinal functions, and may be the cause of stagnation of the blood, irregular digestion and defective blood-supply. Among persons, largely engaged in mental work, such as students and civil service officers their complaints are frequently associated with nervous disorders, head-aches, groundless depression, exaggeration of trifling indisposition etc. *Long continued walking* and *standing* hamper the return of the blood from the lower limbs to the heart and causes for instance in the case of waiters or washerwomen swellings of the feet and ankles, varicose veins or ulcers on the lower limbs (cf. § 107).

§ 174. **Influence of the weather. Effect of very great heat.** Among peasants, agricultural laboures, coachmen, railway workmen, sailors and other persons, much exposed to influences of the weather in their occupations, especially among workmen in underground work, who sometimes are compelled to stand for days in water, diseases of the respiratory organs and rheumatic pains are frequent. Blacksmiths, workmen in foundries, stokers and glass-blowers frequently suffer from skin diseases in consequence of the radiating heat of the furnaces before which they work. Such external influences are borne however by the majority of persons, exposed to them without injury, because the human body becomes inured to them and, as it is said, „hardened" to them.

§ 175. **Dust disease.** In some industries the workmen are compelled to inhale dust, which according to its nature may injure the health in different ways. Soft kinds of dust are least injurious, when they are not mixed with poisonous substances and are not polluted by germs of disease. The coal-dust inhaled by the coalheaver, the soot by the chimney sweep, the graphite dust by the lead pencil-maker und moulder produce troubles in the respiratory organs only very seldom. On the other hand the *diseases of the teeth*, so frequently found among bakers and confectioners are ascribed to the inhaling of *flour-dust*, which remains in the interstices and hollow parts of the teeth, is converted into sugar by the action of the saliva and forms a favourable feeding-ground for the germs of fermentation and bacteria.

To the *dust* of establishments for *polishing glass*, *metal* and *stone* the origin of many lung diseases is due; for the sharp edges and points of the hard glass, metal and stone produce injuries in the side of the branches of the windpipe and lung vesicles which become the inlets for inhaled disease germs.

The nature of some trades brings with it the danger, that the particles of dust in the material to be manufactured are mixed with *infectious substances*, which pass into the workman's body not only by his breath, but also with his food, and may produce illness. Disease germs adhere very tenaciously to *rags, bed-fealhers* etc. which have been used by sick persons; therefore the sorters in paper-works and shoddy-factories are exposed to contagious diseases; and it has been proved that small-pox has been communicated to workers in bed-feather factories in the course of their occupation. The making-up of *hides* and *hair* of animals, who succumbed to *anthrax* have sometimes caused cases of this dangerous illness.

§ 176. **Noxious gases.** In some trades occupied with the manufacture of *poisonous substances* the workmen may suffer injury from inhaling poisonous dust, due to the improper arrangement of the working plant. More frequently however the air of the work-rooms becomes dangerous through contamination with *noxious or poisonous gases*. Thus, bleachers, straw-workers, persons engaged in the manufacture of alum, glass, ultramarine, sulphuric acid and white lead are often exposed to the inhalation of sulphurous acid gas. Similarly, hydrochloric acid gas is produced in soda-works, chloride gas in the manufacture of chloride of lime and in quick-bleaching processes. The employés in gas-works, as well as those engaged in laying-down and repairing gas pipes run various risks from coal-gas, and workers in mines and tunnels are in danger from mining and subterranean gases.

§ 177. **Poisoning by metals or Phosphorus.** In the manufacture of metals poisonous effects may occur not only from inhalation of fumes, but also by poisonous substances adhering to the hands being conveyed to the mouth together with the food or otherwise. In this way arise *mercurial poisonings* among mirror-platers; *lead poisoning* among compositors, house painters and lacquerers using lead colours; among potters and workers in white-lead factories; *arsenical poisoning* among persons employed in making and using arsenical colours, such as Schweinfurth-green, and in the manufacture of artificial flowers. Similarly among those engaged in phosphorus-work, and especially among workmen, employed in making matches, tipped with white phosphorus the *phosphoric fumes* produce bad teeth leading to *caries* in the jaw. Fortunately these matches have been replaced lately by the so-called Swedish matches, which are manufactured by means of a less dangerous process.

§ 178. **Accidents.** In some trades *injuries* sometimes are caused in the working of machines, circular saws, flywheels, electric conductors with high tension etc. Explosions may happen in the manufacture and use of gunpowder and other explosives in the combustion of fire damp and on many other occasions.

§ 179. **Precautionary measures against accidents during**

IV. Profession and business.

work. In order to *reduce* the *business injuries* to health and accidents arising from the risks mentioned in the preceding paragraphs to the lowest degree possible many *laws* and *police regulations* have been passed. Frequently the *carelessness* or want of caution of the injured workman was the cause of the injury. In face of such occurrences it cannot be too often and strongly urged, that it is one of the duties, attached to every occupation or work to be informed thoroughly of the dangers surrounding it, and to comply strictly with the rules in regard to conduct and precaution.

According to the *trade law* the owners of factories have the duty to arrange and keep the workrooms, trade appliances, machines and tools in such order, that the workmen should be protected against dangers to life and health in so far as the charakter of the trade permits. Especially care should be taken to provide sufficient light, air-space and ventilation; removal of dust vapours and gases arising, and of the refuse in the course of the manufacturing of the goods. The owner should also provide all appliances for the protection of the workpeople against contact with the machinery, against all other dangers, arising from working in a factory, especially against a conflagration in the factory. The Federal Council has passed laws with regard to all kinds of factory work, especially those, which endanger in a peculiar manner the life and health of the workers (see above mentioned trades). The *Accident-prevention regulations* can be passed by the committees of the workmen themselves according to the *General Accident-insurance laws* (for workmen) of $\frac{6^{th} \text{ July } 1884}{30^{th} \text{ July } 1900}$ and should be confirmed by the *Imperial Insurance* Department (for workmen). The committee of the workmen have the right to superintend the execution of all the regulation in force with regard to the safety of the workmen.

In spite of the above mentioned regulations of a *preventive* character only too many injuries to health occur in the various trades. But there are in the German Empire at present laws in force, tending to alleviate and to compensate in some degree at least the consequences of these injuries. By the imperial laws of $\frac{10 \text{ April } 1892}{30 \text{ June } 1900}$ referring to the *insurance of workpeople during illness,* the law about *insurance against accidents* of $\frac{6 \text{ July } 1884}{30 \text{ June } 1900}$ and the *insurance law for invalids* of 13 July 1899 *a compulsory insurance of workpeople against illness, accidents during time of work and incapacity to work (invalid, old age)* is now introduced in Germany. The workman is saved from the workhouse (a pauper's institution) by law during the time, when he is temporarily prevented to work, and when by age he is totally incapacitated to work.

At present in Germany all persons, male and female engaged for wages or salary up to 2000 Mark yearly in any trade or profession (about nine million persons in number) are *compulsorily insured against sickness*. The insurance of domestic servants and agricultural labourers is still left to municipal or local laws (but an Imperial Law is in preparation). Each person insured receives in case of sickness medical attendance and all the other necessaries, for instance spectacles, trusses etc. free, gratis; if he is incapacitated from work, he receives at least half the usual or average day's wage for each working day, that he is invalided. These advantages continue during thirteen weeks, if the illness lasts so long. A sum is paid besides to relatives in case of death. The insurance against sickness is carried out by the sick-clubs, each trade or profession or occupation possessing one club. (The Employer pays one third, the employés two thirds of the premium.) 2000 Mark = about £ 100 = 500 Dollars.

The insurance against accidents is far more widespread than the insurance against sickness. *All* persons (about eighteen millions) engaged in industrial works, agriculture, in dangerous trades; artisans, sailors, small offices employes and small contractors (about 4 millions small landowners) are by public law entitled to this *accident insurance, even if the victim himself or a third party* caused the accident. All *sudden occurences*, connected with the industry and the work in which the victim in employed are considered as *accidents;* not however including results, gradually produced by long-continued employment, e. g. in mercurial looking-glass factories, match factories, lead factories etc. (Laws of $\frac{6\text{th July }1884}{30\text{th June }1900}$ cf. § 177). Accidents insurance guarantees *compensation* to the injured person. This compensation consists 1st in defraying all costs of recovery, as well as in a fixed income in money (Rente) called *accident-Rente* for the whole period during which the injured is not capable to work. The *Rente* is to be calculated up to $\frac{2}{3}$ of the yearly average earnings or salary. These payments do not begin until the 14th week after the accident occurred; up to which time the injured receives *compensation* in virtue of the *insurance* against *sickness*. If death results from the accident, the relatives receive money to defray the costs of burial, and the widow (until she remarries) and the children up to their 15th year of age receive annuities. The costs of the accidents insurance is borne *exclusively* by the *employers*; they alone have to form the *trade associations* for the purpose of insuring their workmen against accidents. The workmen contribute nothing to this fund.

The third of these Imperial insurance laws is the "*Invaliden*" *insurance law* of 13th July 1899. It exacts that incapacity for work, resulting from age (seventy years) and not from temporary illness or accidents, is provided for in the following manner. This law applies to all workmen in all branches of trade, inclusive apprentices and domestic servants, officials etc. earning less than 2000 Mark (about 12 million persons). The benefit of this law, an *annuity* of about 150 Mark a year, according to wages and number of years, the insured person has contributed, accrues particularly to those incapacitated from labour by accidents outside their trade, or by diseases gradually contracted in their occupations. The German Empire contributes to each annuity the sum of 50 Mark, while the rest is paid by the employer and the workman ind equal shares.

§ 180. Statistics of illnesses and deaths in different trades and occupations.

To obtain a certain basis for the measures, to be taken to prevent, or to diminish the injuries to health in various occupations, it is necessary to get reliable statistical tables. By learning the character and frequency of injuries to health and accidents in any given branch of work, we learn to appreciate the danger of that labour and of the means to be adopted for lessening or removing it. Different occupations can be compared with one another only by selecting from each as many persons as possible, possessing the same physical constitution, age, mode of life, housing and keeping them under observation for years. It is not however enough to discover that there are less cases of sickness among a thousand blacksmith, than among a thousand shoemakers of the same age during the same period in order to conclude therefrom, that shoemaking is a less healthy trade than that of a blacksmith. It should be taken into consideration, that as a rule stronger persons, who have more power of resistance, become blacksmith than shoemakers. Generally one may consider as doubtless according to the experience, gained up to the present, that working in closed rooms, filled with dust produces more sickness and more cases of death, unless special precautions are taken, than labour in a pure dust-free atmosphere and particularly than work in the open air.

In the meantime statistics of mortality in certain occupations still form the most valuable standard for estimating the dangers to health connected with them. Thus in England for men between the ages of twenty-five and forty-five the smallest mortality was found among clergymen, gardeners and farmers; on the other hand the highest mortality among public-house proprietors and all persons engaged in work in public-houses, filecutters, miners in tin-mines, brewers etc. Relatively rarely succumb fishermen and agricultural labourers workers to consumption; more frequently tailors and printers, compositors. A very high mortality is found among people without a regular permanent trade, as for instance pedlars and similar occupations; but this may perhaps be explained by the fact, that among the latter class there are to be found many weakly persons, who were unable to adopt any heavy work on account of bodily defects or illness.

D. Dangers to health from external influences.

I. Injuries to health from weather and climate.

§ 181. The cause and various classes of colds. Besides the circumstances, mentioned in previous chapters, which can become injurious to health, there are many external causes, independent of the circumstances and mode of life of the individual which may cause an illness to break out.

The influence of the weather on our health is unmistakable. In *hot weather* the skin presents a ruddy appearance and a moist character. The small skin-glands, expanding under the influence of the heat absorb more blood; larger quantities of perspiration are exuded, by the evaporation of which heat is withdrawn from the body. The increased secretion of fluid from the skin causes a greater feeling of thirst and a decrease in the secretions of the kidneys; the urine becomes darker, containing less water. As however the diffusion of heat from the body is still less, than with a cold temperature, excessive accumulation of heat in the body is prevented by lessening the production of heat. Accordingly a diminution in our desire for food and a certain reluctance for muscular work sets in.

In *cold weather* the pores of the skin contract, the exudation of sweat is less, the urine secretion becomes more plentiful, and the colour of the urine is paler. The relatively large quantities of heat, given off to the surrounding colder air must be replaced in the body. Accordingly, the craving for food increases in general, especially preferred is certain food containing fat and carbo-hydrates. By an increase of the activity of the muscles (movements) heat is also produced.

Although the body is capable of adapting itself to the temperature of its surroundings in the manner described, still

I. Injuries to health from weather and climate. 171

higher and lesser degrees of heat and cold are unpleasantly felt. Moreover dryness and dampness of the atmosphere (cf. § 35) as well as variations in its pressure are felt by us. Lastly wind and wet destroy our comfort. Such feelings make us believe, that changes of weather are also causes of injury to our health. Besides, experience teaches us, that persons engaged in occupations more particularly exposed to wind and weather frequently suffer from the same diseases, which appear in the case of other persons after a violent chill or wetting. Such maladies are commonly called *colds*, and among then in particular all acute pains are popularly included; as acute and chronic *rheumatism of the joints*, muscular rheumatism, painful nervous disorders, e. g. face ache and sciatica. Many disorders of the digestive organs, combined with diarrhœa and the so-called *catarrhs* of the respiratory organs are reckoned as colds. The latter, catarrh generally attacks the air-passages, nose, throat, larynx and the windpipe with its branches; it may also lead to inflammation of the lungs and the pleura, and may involve the ears and eyes. These disorders are first seen as redness, caused by an increased blood supply and in swelling of the mucous membrane, which according to the part affected produces sneezing, coughing, intolerance of light, dryness in the throat, hoarseness etc. Soon an increase in the secretion of mucus takes place, plainly noticeable in the mucous membrane of the nose and the throat, and the "dry" catarrh of the beginning of the disorder becomes softer; ("dissolves itself" as it is popularly called) as a result coughing becomes easier and expectoration more plentiful. In lighter attacks the former state of the mucous membrane is restored by proper treatment of the person affected; frequently however the symptoms of the catarrh are accompanied by fever-heat, pains and other disorders; sometimes even dangerous complications may follow a catarrh.

§ 182. **Precautions against "colds".** Although undoubtedly the disorders mentioned above are to a great extent due and caused by the influence of the weather, yet other circumstances are as a rule necessary to produce them. The exaggerated fear of wind, cold and wet and of every harmless draught, which is partly based upon antiquated medical views, is frequently too far-fetched and is often the occasion of injudicious conduct with many people. It is of course advisable to wear protective warm clothing in cold, wind and heavy rain, and to exchange wet clothing against dry as quick as possible; still precautions against cold should not prevent us in remaining in the open air, or insisting upon adequate provision for the ventilation of closed rooms, constantly occupied. The body is rendered effeminate by too warm clothing or too anxious avoiding of the open cool air, and is deprived of the opportunity of becoming inured to the influence of the weather. Thus the capacity of accomodating the body to changes of temperature ceases and the individual becomes more easily the victim of a "cold", against which judicious hardening of the body would have protected him.

§ 183. **Frost-bites.** Another group of maladies, due to the influence of the weather are *frost-bites* of different degrees, whose lightest form is presented by the well-known troublesome chillblains. Frequently their origin is favoured by partial stoppage of the circulation of the blood, e. g. under too closely fitting gloves or tight boots.

The parts of the body, affected by severe frost-bites become first cold, stiff and pallid like a corpse; blisters form on the skin, and finally the frozen members become perfectly dead; as it is commonly called, they become "gangrenous".

The portions of the body which are not moved during intense cold are most exposed to the effects of frost, and therefore the uncomfortable frosty sensation appears soonest on the nose and ears. Benumbing of the limbs occurs especially among persons, who lie down to sleep in the open air during the winter; death from cold may result from the effects of very severe cold. In cold weather we should therefore keep constantly moving and above all should not give in in the open air to the feeling of weariness and craving for sleep.

§ 184. **Treatment of frost bitten persons.** As the body as a rule sinks into an apparently lifeless condition previous to actual death from cold, it is our duty to make efforts at once to resuscitate those who appear to be frozen dead (cf. § 238). The frozen person is accordingly brought into an unheated room, his clothes removed and his body covered with snow, or laid into a tub with cold water, as quick warming would be injurious. The stiff body is then well rubbed with snow or wet cloth, but care should be taken in all treatments of frozen persons not to injure the limbs stiffened by the frost and particularly not to break them. When the limbs become flexible again, the pallor disappears, and bodily heat returns, the patient should be laid in an unwarmed bed, and there submitted by his helpers to a course of artificial breathing (§ 239) until he can breathe regularly without assistance. An effort should also be made to pour tepid tea or coffee and afterwards wine or brandy down his throat. Only, when consciousness, warmth, mobility and respiration are completely restored, can the convalescent be brought into a warm room and be placed in a warm bed.

Similar treatment is adopted for single parts of the body when frozen, as for the whole body. They are to be protected from being warmed too quickly and should be rubbed assiduously with snow or damp cloths, but not so roughly as to remove the skin; because in that case sores are formed which take a long time to heal. The parts of the body affected should then be covered with antiseptic cottonwool or clean linen, after having saturated the bandages with good oil or smeared with ointment.

§ 185. **Heat-stroke; sun-stroke: lightning stroke.** Excessive heat also brings with it serious dangers to health, as it may cause *heat-stroke*, which frequently terminates fatally. Attacks of this nature occur most easily, when the air is almost motionless and is saturated with moisture. The evaporation of sweat then proceeds slowly, and consequently the body is not sufficiently cooled. In dry atmosphere the skin exhalations become too small, if the water, withdrawn from the body by perspiration is not replaced from time to time by drinking. If in either of these two cases the air is too warm to effect a proper cooling of the body, and if the heat, generated in the body is not diffused sufficiently, then the temperature of the blood increases, attains a hight, which is usually only found among persons suffering from fever (§ 193) and finally produces the dangerous malady heat-stroke.

Heat-stroke most frequently occurs in the case of persons, who undertake long marches in closed, compact masses, e. g. soldiers. Here much heat is produced by muscular exertion, while the surface of each individual's body is less accessible to cooling by the air, on account of the closely marching ranks. The face of the person, suffering from heat-stroke becomes red, his head becomes giddy, interest in conversation disappears, no answer is given to questions and the man keeps marching with the others as if in a dream. If the soldier at this stage of the attack is removed from the closed volumn, and if the diffusion of heat from the surface of his body is rendered easier, and the heat produced by marching interrupted, the imminent collapse passes over quickly as a rule, especially, when cooling drinks are supplied and the skin of the whole body sprinkled with water. But if the person attacked continues marching in closed ranks he loses consciousness, his pulse becomes weak and irregular, breathing only takes place superficially and finally ceases and the man sinks down in convulsions.

In the German army, the officers, non-commissioned officers and men are afforded an opportunity by frequently reiterated instructions of recognising and averting in time the danger of an attack of heat-stroke.

In the case of an attack of heat-stroke medical aid should be procured as quickly as possible. Until the physician arrives, the patient is to be treated in the same manner like a person, who has swooned (§ 237). It is especially necessary to restore respiration (should it have failed) by artificial means (§ 239) and to apply ice or cold water bandages to the hot head, and, if possible cool the body by bathing or at least sprinkling with cold water.

A malady, similar to heat-stroke is *sun-stroke;* which may affect even persons resting and not engaged in muscular efforts by the direct radiation of a hot noon-day sun on the head. The heating of the head causes a rush of blood to the brain, and in consequence headache, giddiness, swimming before the eyes, nausea, vomiting and faintness set in. In severe cases it may lead to convulsions, raving and even death. Persons, afflicted with sun-stroke should be brought into the shade as quickly as possible, and treated in the same manner as for heat-stroke.

Similar assistance should be given to persons struck by lightning. The latter are usually found in an apparently lifeless condition but frequently recover under the influence of efforts made to resuscitate them. Sometimes loss of power of the limbs remains but this also mostly disappears under proper treatment.

§ 186. Climate and seasons. Different diseases have been proved to owe their origin to the climate and to the season of the year. Thus consumption is found preeminently among people, exposed to a severe climate, and other chest diseases, such as catarrh and inflammation of the lungs occur most frequently among us in the winter and spring. Yellow fever, dysentery and malaria are either exclusively or to a very large extent confined to tropical regions. Enteric fever and diarrhœa in children are observed more frequently in hot seasons than at other times. Many diseases peculiar to foreign countries run a comparatively mild course with the natives, while they are more serious for strangers, travelling through the country, who have not become acclimatized or accustomed to the new climatic conditions. Anyone, who, when changing climate does not adopt diligently a regular mode of life, or omits to adapt himself to the changed conditions according to the advice of experienced and intelligent persons, renders his body susceptible to such diseases, just as on the other hand, he, who in irrational exaggerated zeal suddenly changes completely the habits, necessary for his well-being also becomes an easy victim to disease germs.

II. Infectious diseases.

a) In general.

§ 187. Nature and manner of spreading infectious diseases. Climate and season, in spite of their undeniable influence on the origin of many diseases are in reality not the direct cause of them; they only supply the conditions favourable to disease, either by promoting the vitality and growth of disease germs, or by diminishing the power of the human body of resisting these germs. The essential cause of many diseases, and particularly of most that are connected with climate and season is to be thought in living small microbes, which penetrating into our body taint or "infect" it. All diseases, which owe their origin in this way to a communicable disease germ are called *infectious diseases*.

The infectious diseases can be transferred to a human being either direct by tainted persons and their excretions or by means of healthy persons or animals (e. g. flies) who propagate only the infectious germs; moreover by means of animals (e. g. rats in cases of plague, mosquitoes in cases of malaria) who have in their bodies suitable conditions for the propagation of the virus; finally by means of inanimate things, such as water, dust, food, clothes, linen etc.) which contain the communicable disease germ or *virus*. In most infectious diseases we have to consider with regard to its propagation the direct communication or transfer as well as the indirect communication.

§ 188. **Disease germs.** For a number of infectious diseases we have succeded in obtaining the disease germs in the form of certain minute micro-organisms, already referred to repeatedly. In each of these diseases organisms, peculiar to each were found in the blood, the tissue, the juices and the excreta of the body; and these organisms were invariably absent in the case of healthy or differently affected persons. We have succeeded in rearing some of these germs on artificially prepared feeding grounds, e. g. meat-broth, thickened by the addition of gelatine, and by transferring these artificially bred germs to animals, have been able to produce in the latter the symptoms, peculiar to the disease in question. Sometimes by accident, imprudence or experiments, which courageous savants have made on themselves, it has been proved that artificially-bred germs produce sickness in men. These advances, made by science in the knowledge of disease date only from the last few years and are due in the first line to *R. Koch;* Thus is has been shown, how important a thorough investigation of the vital conditions of these micro-organisms is in order to understand and to overcome infectious diseases.

The majority of the living organisms, hitherto described as disease germs, are of a vegetable nature and belong to the family of the fissiparous fungi. Since many of them possess the form of short rods, they are called "bacteria" from the greek word for rod. They appear sometimes singly, sometimes in groups, or arranged in the form of a chain. According to shape they are either rod-like (bacilli) or spherical (cocci); some have a crooked form (comma-bacilli or vibriones); others the form of a screw or a worm (spirilli); many kinds possess more or less active movements of their own, others are motionless. The propagation of bacteria is affected by fission; the young organisms, thus produced grow to the size of the parent bacteria and then in their turn divide themselves. This process is repeated so rapidly, that milliards of micro-organisms may be produced within a few hours from a small number. Many kinds form "spores", permanent structures, as within the individual spore a spherical or egg-shaped body is formed, which is preserved in the fission of the original parent organism and is able to offer greater resistance to the effect of heat and cold and also to many substances, fatal to bacteria. If a spore of this kind, which is somewhat similar to the seed of a plant is brought under conditions, favourable to its vitality, it grows to the size of the parent bacterium. Disease germs, which otherwise can thrive only inside the body may therefore retain their capacity development

II. Infectious diseases.

outside the body in the shape of spores, and may reproduce themselves as soon as they penetrate into another body. All bacteria are so small, that they can be recognized only, when greatly magnified, and nearly all are particularly colourless; they are destinguished however in great part by the fact, that they can absorb and tenaciously retain certain colouring substances. Therefore, if a fragment of animal tissue, coagulated blood, etc. is treated with such a colouring substance and then washed, the bacteria alone remain coloured in the colourless tissue. In this way the bacteria can be more easily recognised under the microscope than in their natural condition.

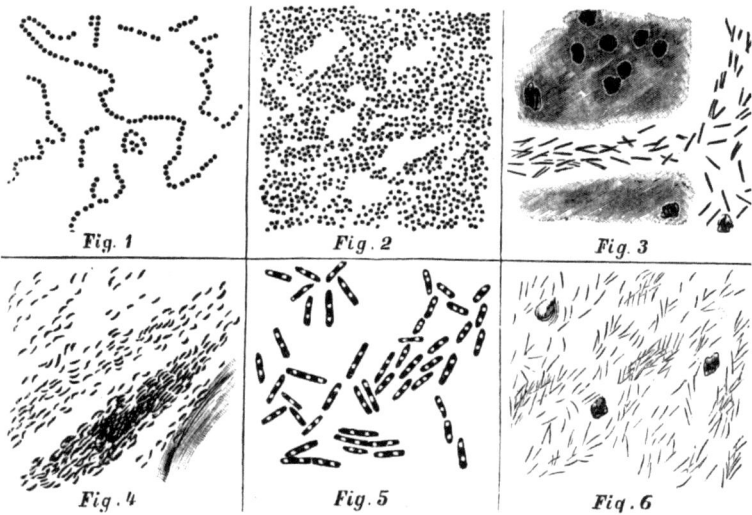

Fig. 42. Diagrammatic representation of Bacteria. (Greatly magnified.)
1. Cocci in chain form. *2.* Cocci in groups. *3.* Bacilli in a capillary vessel. *4.* Comma-bacilli. *5.* Bacilli with spores. *6.* Very fine bacilli.

The bacteria multiply in certain liquids to such a degree, that they are visible to the naked eye as a cloudy discoloration. On a solid substance, on which they grow they form by their growth colonies, each consisting of millions of single organisms, but which appear to the unaided eye merely as minute drops, knobs, or slight protuberances. If, for instance a boiled potatoe is cut in two and exposed for some minutes to the air, and then placed under a glass shade, such colonies of bacteria may be observed on the cut surface after twenty four hours which have been developed from single bacteria deposited by the atmosphere.

By their growth the bacteria alter the composition of the feeding ground, as they withdraw from it certain substances, necessary for their structure and thus various chemical combinations may arise. In this way they cause many processes of fermentation and decomposition by action, similar to the yeast fungi, already mentioned. Many species of bacteria also separate poisonous substances from their feeding ground (§ 61) which may have even in very small quantities fatal effects on the human body; other bacteria contain poison themselves. Thus by the nature and vital functions of the bacteria is explained the injurious effect on the human system peculiar to many of them. The illnesses, produced by bacteria originate, according to our present information either in the destruction of the tissues serving as their feeding ground or in the poisonous substances separated by them or in their own poisonous action. Some infectious diseases are ascribed to activity of certain animal micro-organisms (Fig. 42).

Among the incalculably great number of bacilli only relatively few species are however injurious to health. The human body contains permanently inumerable small living organisms, which are partly harmless spores and partly assist in certain bodily functions e. g. digestion. Other germs are unable to exist inside the human body and perish as soon as they are introduced with food or otherwise. Lastly; there are also micro-organisms, which are not properly disease producers, but which may be injurious to health, if they pass into the body in large quantities, or have acquired abnormal qualities; among these are included some germs of decomposition and many bacteria, present even in the healthy intestines.

§ 189. **Preliminary conditions of infection.** The disease germs require certain predisposing conditions in order to be capable to produce their peculiar effects. The frequent appearance of *infectious diseases* in certain places *(endemics)* or the sudden rapid spreading of such diseases *(epidemics)* their subsequent extinction and the immunity of other districts cannot be exclusively explained by the presence, absence or introduction of the corresponding micro-organisms. The numerous special circumstances, not yet completely investigated, which promote in endemics or epidemics the spread of disease germs 1^t at certain times, 2^d in certain places and 3^d among certain persons or classes of persons are provisionally described as 1^t temporal, 2^d local and 3^d personal "predispositions". A *temporal predisposition* is afforded by the action of the weather, such as abnormal heat, moisture of the atmosphere, which temporarily provides conditions favourable to the spread and virulence of the disease germs. Many epidemics find a *local predisposition* among others in the neighbourhood of swamps in unhealthy or overcrowded dwellings, in a bad water-supply and in defective arrangements for the removal of refuse.

The importance of *personal* or *individual "predisposition"* is very great. It is observed in times of epidemics, that only a limited portion of the population, exposed to the danger of infection, suffer; and some families are unusually susceptible to certain diseases of an infectious nature. The predisposition to many illnesses — e. g. consumption — is transmitted from the parents to the children and to the grand-children. Although in getting or not getting these infectious diseases chance infection plays a great part, and though the immunity of certain persons such as physicians during epidemics can easily be explained by their taking proper precaution, still we must assume an immunity in many men and a predisposition in others towards infectious diseases. The immunity from an infectious disease can be innate or acquired, but may be lost again under certain conditions, for instance in consequence of hardship or want of nourishment. It is known, that most people, after recovering from an infectious disease, for instance small-pox or measles are not attacked a second time by the same disease.

Recently it has been found, that the inoculation of the "serum" of the blood of animals, which have suffered certain infectious diseases, or which by certain methods of treatment have become immune to certain forms of illness, gives other animals or men the power of withstanding those diseases and sometimes indeed of becoming cured, when already infected with the disease. Efforts are being made at present to realize these observations for combating infectious diseases (cf. § 206).

§ 190. Preventive measures against infectious diseases. The efforts towards *warding off infectious diseases* had already led to good results before the germs of disease in the microorganisms had become know. In former times epidemics wrougth far greater devastation than at present. In the fourteenth century the black death is reported to have carried off 25 millions of people i. e. about the fourth part of all people then living in Europe. Small-pox and typhus alone caused regularly more deaths than all infectious diseases at present. Especially the number of cases of infectious diseases diminished considerably, where attention was paid to the rules of hygiene.

In the Prussian army in 1869 22 216 soldiers were attacked by infectious diseases; after ten years the number fell to

11467; ten years further the number of cases was only 4695; and in 1895 only 4077 soldiers were attacked by infectious disease; although the numerical strength of the Prussian army has been considerably increased since 1870.

Munich was formerly considered as very unhealthy; for between 1850 and 1860 213, in 1858 as many as 334 and between 1867 and 1875 130 persons per 100000 of the inhabitants yearly died of typhoid fever. Upon the advice of von Pettenkofer it was decided to improve the sanitary conditions of the town. Care was taken to have a suitable removal of refuse; private slaughter-houses were abolished altogether and good drinking water was procured by obtaining spring water brought into town through an aquaeduct. Since then the number of cases of death diminished constantly; already between 1876 and 1878 only 42 died on the average yearly and from 1893 to 1899 only 5 persons of 100000 die on an average yearly in Munich from typhoid fever. Similar results in respects to the decrease of infectious disease have been shown in many other German towns; such as Berlin and Dantzig in consequence of sanitary improvements.

As the power of resisting infection in the individual is increased by proper mode of life and suitable nourishment, so an efficacious means of combating infectious diseases is found in the healthy arrangemont of communities. Nevertheless man is not sufficiently protected against infection without additional safeguards.

§ 191. **Combating infectious diseases.** In the chapter on commerce we have already described the means adopted for preventing the spread of infection from place to place and from country to country. In order to be able to suppress effectually an epidemic, that has broken out in a town or country, it is necessary that every case of it should be promptly reported to the authorities; furthermore each case should be supervised so as not to become the starting-point of further infection. The essential means for these purposes are: 1st the *duty imposed* on doctors, the relatives of the sick, or other people responsible for them, of *notifying the illness*; 2^d the *isolation* of the sick (and if necessary of persons having intercourse with him) from the healthy population; and 3^d the *destruction* or *disinfection* of the disease germs in the excreta of the sick, in their linen and clothing and in all objects, to which the infectious matter might adhere.

For destroying disease germs the best means is burning; but such an extreme measure is only resorted to, when disinfection would be too costly in comparison to the value of the tainted object. A disinfecting process should be effective, cheap, harmless to the objects treated by it and free from danger to the persons entrusted with its execution. Disinfection is effective, if it destroys the infectious matter or renders it innocuous, a goal, that can be attained only under the guidance of skilled persons.

The following processes are used for disinfection.

1. Heating by steam. For this process are used either movable, steam-producing apparatus which are brought from place to place like locomotives, or stationary boilers, erected in special disinfecting rooms. Steam apparatus, from which a reliable result is to be expected should be examined by competent persons and attended to by trained workers. When well-constructed and properly-fed ones are used, the steaming process destroys disease-germs with great certainty and possesses the advantage of not injuring most objects. However, leather objects, furs, india rubber goods, glued, polished or veneered articles, some metal wares and many kinds of furniture are rendered valueless by it and hence should not be disinfected in this way. The finer articles of clothing require mending and pressing after the action of the steam. Cloth or linen garments, which have been defiled with blood, matter or human excreta should be washed before being placed in the steam apparatus, or otherwise permanent stains are usually left behind. All objects, disinfected by steam are benefited by being protected from the water deposited during cooling by means of coverings of sacking etc.

2. Boiling. The objects to be disinfected are placed in boiling water, to which some soda has been added. The process is easily carried out, and when continued long enough produces reliable results; it is however inapplicable to many objects. It is most suitable for underclothing, small metallic objects, utensils etc.

3. Chemical treatment. a) Solution of carbolic soap. To a solution, consisting of 3 parts of soft-soap and 100 parts of water 5 parts of commercial carbolic acid are added, while the solution is being constantly stirred. Linen and other suitable material are steeped for a long time in the solution; wooden articles, floors, the walls of rooms, shoes and other leather articles are washed with it. Sometimes the soap solution without the carbolic acid is sufficient. The smell, caused by the acid is removed from the disinfected objects by washing or airing.

b) *Whitewash.* This is prepared by mixing one part of broken, well-burnt lime with 4 parts of water. It is best carried out in the following manner. In the preparing vessel only a small portion of the water is first poured; the lime is added, which absorbs the water and in a short time is reduced to powder, steam and heat being thereby produced. Then the rest of the water is added, while the contents are kept stirred. The disinfecting fluid, prepared in this way should be kept in well-closed vessels and be shaken before being used. In handling whitewash care should be taken that none of it is allowed to come in contact with the eyes, as it is a corrosive fluid, highly injurious to the eyes.

Whitewash is particularly suitable for disinfecting the excreta of the sick. When thoroughly mixed in equal proportions with the latter it kills the disease germs or micro-organisms therein in a short time. It is also used with advantage for disinfecting the sick-room by washing or painting the walls and floors admitting such treatment, and repeating the process after a short interval.

4. Beating, brushing, airing, sunning. This treatment is applied to objects, which would be rendered useless by boiling or wetting, as well as to objects, which would be unsuitable for disinfection by steam, e. g. many upholstered articles. The process suffices for the removal of certain disease germs; it is not be relied on however.

5. Other means. Some other disinfecting processes are used, according to the circumstances of the case. Thus, a number of chemical substances, e. g. corrosive sublimate (a mercurial compound) formaldehyde, thymole, chloride of lime and of zinc are useful means of disinfection in certain cases. Some of them are specially suited for destroying diseased matter on the hands and other parts of the body, but in such cases a thorough soaplather with a brush should precede disinfection. The whole body is most thoroughly disinfected by a bath with plentiful use of soap. Infectious substances are removed from wall paper by rubbing them with breadcrumbs, which should be burnt after being used; or the wallpaper is entirely removed, to that the walls may be whitewashed. The joinings of the boards in the floor should be sprinkled with the disinfecting fluids; sometimes it is necessary to remove the entire dust from under the floor (cf. § 115).

Formaldehyde is a gaseous body, which is easily soluble in water, and is employed in aqueous solution as well as in the gaseous state. Recently several methods have become known for the employment of gaseous formaldehyd for disinfection by all of which only the disease germs on easily attainable surfaces are killed with certainty; e. g. on wallpaper (tapestry). Woven materials (cloaks, quilts), or porous objects are not pierced through by the gas. A disinfection with formaldehyde should be only undertaken with the advise of a physician and under his supervision. Unfortunately, some unreliable modes of disinfection are still largely employed. Among them are the treatment of the object with sulphate of iron or of copper, or with sulphuric acid. Even fumigating with chlorine gas and spraying with diluted carbolic acid are often insufficient, because the disinfectants are not used in sufficient quantities.

The manner, extent and duration of disinfection should in every case be decided by an expert preferably by the doctor, and the execution of the process should be placed under medical supervision, so far as it cannot be entrusted to special disinfecting works. Establishments of this kind are to be found in many large towns and in many country districts. The skilled staff attend with the necessary appliances at the house of the patient in order to disinfect it, and the immovable objects in the dwelling, clothing, bedding, furniture and utensils from the sick room and other movable objects are taken away in well-closed carts and brought back to the house twentyfour hours laters after complete disinfection.

Abuse of disinfection frequently occurs, especially in times of epidemics. Travellers and their luggage are sprinkled with disinfectants; the streets and various objects, which cannot remotely be suspected of being infected with disease germs are sprinkled with the same fluids. Apart from the fact, that such a proceeding is unnecessarily molesting and occasions a boundless waste of disinfectants, it has the particular disadvantage of giving the people the erroneous belief, that they are thus secured against the epidemics. Thus frequently then the real means from preventing the spread of the disease are easily overlooked and relying on the efficacy of the disinfectants *cleanliness* is neglected, which is in every case *more useful, than inefficient disinfection.*

§ 192. **Course of illnesses, arising from infection.** The most important condition for combating an infectious disease is the immediate identification of each individual case. It is therefore necessary to be informed, how these diseases usually progress and the manner in which they enter the human body. Although infectious diseases differ in many ways from one another in this respect, still they have much in common as regards their origin, external symptoms and course of development.

The disease germs find their means of ingress into the human body through the larger openings in the body, especially through air and food passages (nose and mouth) or through sores, often through scarcely visible abrasions of the skin and sometimes even through the pores of the skin. Many germs induce changes at the ingress point, or at least within that organ, into which they first pass. Others migrate in the course of the lymph or blood, in order either to multiply there, or carried on by the circulation to settle themselves in other parts of the body. In every case there follows after the ingress of the germs a period time required for their multiplication and for the formation of the poisonous matter, during which the infected person is still apparently healthy;

this *period* is called the "*stage of incubation*" of the disease. Towards the end of this period, which has a different duration for each infectious disease premonitory symptoms of the disease exhibit themselves, such as weariness, loss of appetite, general painful sensations, a feeling of discomfort etc. Next ensues the outbreak of the disease, sometimes accompanied by vomiting, chill and shivering, sometimes even to chattering of the teeth.

§ 193. Fever. There is a disorder, peculiar to many infectious diseases which in called *fever*. This is the external expression of a heightened „*Stoffumsatz*", i. e. of a greater combustion in the tissues of the body, and forms in many cases an auxiliary to nature in resisting the disease germs and in destroying their poisonous matter. The most prominent characteristic of fever is the measurable increase in the temperature of the body (cf. § 22). A bloodheat raised to 39.5^0 C. corresponds to a moderate fever, a still greater increase to high fever. The frequency of respiration is increased, as also is the number of pulse-beats, corresponding to a greater activity of the heart; the patient suffers from thirst, perspires sometimes and evacuates only small quantities of a highly red urine, which often leaves a deposit layer. The patient complains of headache, giddiness and vertigo, suffers from delirium, talks wildly, clutches distractedly about him, and wishes to leave the bed. If he is not well watched in such a condition, there is a danger of his injuring himself, falling out of bed, jumping from the window etc.

In some infectious diseases the fever remains at about the same height for several weeks, in others the temperature sinks about 1^0 C. regularly in the morning and rises again in the evening; in others the fever disappears after several hours or in a few days. Increase and decline of the fever sometimes takes place gradually, sometimes quickly. A sudden decline of the fever, generally accompanied by perspiration and refreshing sleep is called a "crisis".

Infectious diseases are either followed by a convalescence, or they leave behind, after having run their course disorders in the functions of special organs, after illness, tedious loss of strength, permanent infirmity, or they end with the death of the person attacked.

b) Some infectious diseases.

§ 194. Acute eruptive diseases. Infectious diseases, which display similarities in their external symptoms, their mode of spreading, and their course are usually combined in groups. Thus *measles, German measles, scarlet fever, small-pox, chicken-pox* and *spotted fever* are collectively described as *acute eruptive diseases*, because all are acutely developed, and are distinguished from others by the appearance of eruptions on the skin. The eruptive diseases named are infectious; they spread themselves usually by direct communication from the sick, but are also communicated by healthy persons, who have come in contact with the patient, or by the cloths, linen etc. worn by the latter. The infectious matter of some of them also adheres to the sickroom and thus may prove dangerous to future occupants. Each of these diseases possesses besides quite a special individual characteristic.

§ 195. Measles and German measles. In *measles*, in ten to fourteen days after infection, an eruption of the skin, in the shape of irregularly round and somewhat raised red spots usually appears along with moderate fever. This eruption is first exhibited on the face, and then spreads quickly over the neck, trunk and limbs, so that the body seems almost spotted with red. Whilst these changes are proceeding, catarrhs develop themselves in different mucous membranes, the eyes become bloodshot, and the lids become half closed. Light is avoided as unendurable; snuffing, coughing and hoarseness are among the ordinary symptoms. When the outbreak has reached its maximum, the fever declines and whilst the rash generally disappears the epidermis is renewed by peeling off.

Measles only seldom attacks the same person twice. It occurs generally in Germany as a children's disease, and generally, since very few escape infection before arriving at maturity. Often games played together with other children, Kindergarten and other schools form the occasion for its transmission. In case the illness is introduced in a family it attacks usually all the children one after another.

Although measles as a rule is cured, especially among children, it is advisable, that a physician should be called in, even for light attacks, and that the patient should never be considered as restored to health sooner than four weeks after the appearance of the disease, for, by imprudent treatment, consequences, sometimes of a serious nature arise out of the catarrhs accompanying the disease viz.: lung disease, with affections of the eyes and ears.

The dissemination of the disease can be prevented by perfect isolation of the patient and by disinfection of their excretions, as well as of the linen, clothing and other articles used by them. Generally the brothers and sisters of such patients are excluded from the public schools by order of the authorities. When measles break out generally among school children, it may become necessary to close the class temporarily or even the entire school. The precautions usually taken to prevent the spread of measles are however generally too late, because the disease is very infectious in its early stages, before the appearance of the rash places its character byond doubt.

German measles is a discase very similar to ordinary measles and according to the opinion of many physicians only a variety of it. It is distinguished from the latter by its milder course especially by an absence or subsidence of catarrhs.

§ 196. **Scarlet fever (Scarlatina).** On an average scarlatina begins from four to eight days after infection, and is usually accompanied by high fever, whose commencement is signalized by shivering or vomiting. The patient complains of swelling of the tonsils, followed by difficulty in swallowing; soon there spreads over the body, usually beginning on the trunk or legs a somewhat uniform, raspberry-coloured rash, and the tongue, when not covered with a white coating also exhibits a raspberry-red colour. After a few days, sometimes even after a few hours, the rash begins to decline, and at the same time in favourable cases the fever disappears. The skin finally undergoes a process of scaling, lasting for several weeks.

In no small number of cases of scarlatina the rash is not completely developed on the surface and then the presence of the disease can only be inferred from the course of the illness and from its resemblance to other cases of scarlatina.

Scarlatina should always be considered a very serious illness; sometimes death occurs even in its early stages: but more frequently it becomes fatal through the diseases, which accompany and follow it. A concomitant disease to be often looked for is an affection of the tonsils, similar to diphteria (§ 206). As resulting diseases, affection of the ears, rheumatism, purulent inflammations of the joints and of the lymphatic glands in the jaws *inflammation of the kidneys* sometimes appear. The latter occurs usually along with dropsical swelling of the skin of the face or legs. The physician may infer its presence from finding albumin and cellular tissue in the urine.

Having regard to these dangers the scarlatina patient must be constantly watched and treated by physicians, and especially should be protected from injurious external influences for several weeks in a uniform temperature. Imprudent conduct, e. g. getting up too soon favours the development of after-diseases, which have often caused death or general debility after apparently light attacks.

Scarlatina mostly attacks in preference children and juvenile persons, but sometimes also attacks adults.

Having regard to the frequently serious course of the disease, every precaution should be taken to prevent its spreading, and greater success may be counted upon by attending to such efforts, than in the case of measles. For, as scarlatina attains its maximum power of contagion only after full development the preventive measures are less liable to be late than with measles. The patients should be strictly isolated. With regard to prevent further spreading of the disease through schools special measures are to be adopted, and the disinfection of the patient's excreta, of the articles, used by him, and of the sick-room appears all the more indispensable, as it is beyond doubt, that the infectious matter can be transmitted by inanimate objects (letters, food, bedding) and adheres for a long period to rooms.

§ 197. **Small-pox.** *Small-pox* as a rule breaks out in from ten to thirteen days after infection. The illness begins with a high fever, great depression, pains in the head, difficulty in swallowing, and shooting pain in the "os sacrum". After a few days red pimples show themselves with an abatement of the fever. They appear first on the face, then on the remaining surface of the body, and on the mucous membranes, and from them peculiarly-shaped pustules, containing a transparent liquid, develop. During the following days the liquid contents become turbid, and when about ten days of the illness have elapsed, begin to assume a purulent character, accompanied by a fresh increase of the fever. Within about twelve days these pustules begin to dry up, with a decline of the accompanying fever, and scabs are formed, which afterwards fall off, leaving behind radiating pocknarbs. When the course of the disease is uninterrupted, six weeks usually elapse since the beginning of the disease until full recovery of the patient.

Small-pox often results fatally, especially when it appears as so-called "black small-box" — i. e. when the contents of the pustules become dark in colour from an admixture of blood, or when affections of the brain, throat, lungs or kidneys supervene. The outbreak of pustules in the eyes may result in complete or partial blindness, their appearance in the organs of hearing may occasion total or partial deafness.

A somewhat less tedious and less violent form than the *true small-pox* is the so-called *false small-pox*, otherwise called "modified" pox or "*varioloid*". The mild aspect of this form should however not be the occasion for carelessness in reference to the preventive measures to be taken against its spreading, as the infection caused by it is the same as that of the true small pox.

Small-pox belongs to the most dreaded of infectious diseases; frequently it carries off more than half of those attacked, and leaves behind it, as a legacy to those, who have escaped death, general debility and infirmity. Moreover the infection is exceptionally easy of transmission, as contagion is communicated not only from one person to another, but is also conveyed by the objects touched by the sick persons and even by currents of air.

In the eighteenth century one tenth of the children and large numbers of grown persons fell victims to small-pox. In vain were attempts made to restrict the ravages of the disease by isolation of those attacked. By means of inanimate objects incapable of disinfection by the measures then in use and through the intercourse of healthy persons with the patients the contagion continued to be carried from the sick-rooms, and caused the most devastating epidemics.

§ 198. Vaccination. Shortly before the end of the eighteenth century the world received in *vaccination* a weapon, by which it was to overcome the terror of this epidemic. In the year 1798 the English physician Jenner published the fact already known for a long time and investigated by him in his home in Gloucestershire; namely that an inoculation with the contents of the poxlike pustules sometimes appearing on cows udders, the so-called "cow-pock" affords a protection against the attack of the genuine small-pox. His investigations were soon confirmed. It was afterwards shown however, that the protection acquired by inoculation gradually decreases, and hence, if the body is to remain permanently safeguarded against small-pox, the protection must be renewed by a repetition of the inoculating process.

The Imperial vaccination Law of 1874 provides, that every child in the calendar year, in which the completion of its first year of existence falls, and every pupil of a school in the year, in which he completes his twelfth year must be vaccinated, unless a previous attack of small-pox insures immunity from a recurrence of the disease. Those liable to military service are revaccinated on entering the army or navy. By the appointment of vaccinating doctors, paid by the Government everybody is afforded an opportunity of obeying the law as to vaccination without any expense.

For the purposes of vaccination the contents of the *cow-pock*, produced in calves by inocculation (*animal lymph*) is almost universally used in Germany, while formerly a preference was shown for inocculation by human pock (*humanized lymph*). The latter process has been abandoned chiefly, because it was feared, that with such lymph, not only the vaccine, but also chance diseases of the person from whom the lymph was derived would by communicated. This danger is excluded by using animal lymph.

The strict supervision of the production of lymph and of the institutions, formed for that purpose, partly under municipal control, is a garantee that the lymph is derived from healthy animals.

Usually the upper arm is selected as the vaccinating spot. The development of the pock follows in five or six days after vaccination, sometimes accompanied by fever and swelling of the neighbouring skin. Children, who have been vaccinated are frequently out of sorts at the time, just as when cutting their teeth, but they soon regain their vivacity.

In the *treatment* of *vaccinated* persons chief attention should be given to cleanliness and to prevent the spot vaccinated from becoming sore. The incisions are closed in a few minutes by a light scurf and thus remain permanently protected from impurities, since the pustules arising afterwards do not open but dry up and scab over. As a rule, it is only necessary that the spot selected should be carefully washed with water and soap before vaccination, and should be subsequently kept covered with clean, not too tight clothes. Children should be kept clean, and should be carefully but thoroughly washed once a day naturally avoiding the pock. Children should be prevented from scratching the spot vaccinated or the pock, as it develops, and also from moving their arms too vigorously. If the spot vaccinated festers notwithstanding these precautions, a bandage should be placed on it by a skilled hand. Covering the sore with dirty bandages, or smearing it with dirty, rancid fat brings the danger with it of an infection of the wound.

In exceptional cases after vaccination skin eruptions or inflamed sores have appeared, such as are associated sometimes with superficial wounds of every kind. These symptoms are almost always to be ascribed to neglect in the treatment of the person vaccinated and can be avoided with a little care. It need not be a cause of surprise; if other diseases of childhood set in some days after vaccination, that an attempt should be made to ascribe to vaccination such chance coincidences.

Since the introduction of the vaccination laws small-pox has become an almost unknown disease in Germany; while it causes yearly considerable loss of life in those neighbouring countries, where compulsory vaccination has as yet not been carried out thoroughly; e. g. in many districts of Austria, Russia, some parts of France and Belgium. The few cases of small pox, still observed annually in Germany are almost all imported from foreign countries, and this explains, why the majority of such cases occur in seaports and frontier towns. Thus between 1886—1897 out of 1179 fatal cases of small-pox in the whole empire 929 took place in seaports and frontier towns. Isolation of persons attacked and careful disinfecting measures should however not be omitted in cases of small-pox despite the protection, afforded to people by vaccination in consideration of the unvaccinated children and of adults, who have not been revaccinated.

§ 199. **Chicken-pox.** A disease, different from the *true* and from the *spurious* small-pox is the so-called *chicken-pox* or *varicella*. It generally attacks children under ten years, is also contagious, and reveals itself by the appearance of small pustules on the face, arms and other parts of the body. The rash disappears in a short time without leaving ony scars behind, and generally in a few days the disease is gone.

§ 200. **Typhus. Spotted fever.** Spotted fever or spotted typhus is also frequently described as war or famine typhus, because the disease has frequently developed and spread in times of famine among the starving population, or in time of war among the troops, weakened by privations and hardships. In Germany during the last century the disease has in an epidemic form visited especially Upper Silesia and East Prussia; but it has been observed also in other parts of the Empire, especially in Central Germany.

The disease runs its course with high fever, and is distinguished by a rash, which appears after the first days of illness, and resembles the rash of measles, but is less diffuse and usually spares the face. The consciousness of the patient is almost always clouded; the fever lasts in favourable cases about two weeks; but $\frac{1}{6}$ or $\frac{1}{7}$ of the patients succumb already before that time; sometimes, illnesses, which supervene afterwards, sometimes cause the death of the patient.

Spotted fever is one of the most easily communicable diseases; the contagious matter can both be transferred from the sick to the healthy and be introduced by inanimate objects. The disease is most frequently spread by tramps, pedlers, beggars and such-like people; its dissemination is to be combated by isolation of the patients and by disinfection.

§ 201. **Remittent Fever.** Together with the spotted fever, the remittent fever and typhoid fever are combined by some experts in a common "group", called *typhoid diseases*, although the three diseases are quite distinct from one another.

Remittent fever, also called remittent typhus is produced by a bacillus of spiral form, which has been known already for some time; it is not a disease, which frequently occurs, but is easily communicated, and exhibits itself in repeated attacks of high fever, each lasting from five to six days. The spread of remittent fever is caused in the same way as spotted fever by wandering people, especially in dirty inns. The preventive measures are the same as for spotted fever.

§ 202. **Typhoid fever.** *Typhoid fever* (known in Germany as "Unterleibstyphus" or "Darmtyphus" or "Typhus") has its name from a greek word, which really means smoke or mist, but metaphorically refers to the state of the patient. Thanks to the improvements in public Hygiene in several large towns in Germany, where formerly numerous cases of illness and death and even widespread epidemics were caused by typhoid fever, this disease has become rarer (cf. § 190) it prevails however unfortunately still in the country and also in many towns. In the twenty years from 1877 to 1896 49948 persons died from typhoid in the towns of Germany, which have populations of not less than 15000, being a yearly average of 2497 death for the whole Empire; since 1877 there has been a steady decline in the number of deaths from typhoid, e. g. in each quinquennium since 1877; so that for the five years from 1887—1891 the yearly average only amounted to 2269 although the population of the towns had increased considerably; in the five years 1892 to 1896 the yearly average of death from typhoid for the whole empire fell to 1666 and in the year 1899 the number of deaths was only 1639.

The infection is mostly propagated by means of the drinking water, frequently also by the milk, used in our households.

The interval between reception of the infectious substance and the outbreak of the disease lasts as a rule from 2 to 3 weeks, sometimes even 4 weeks. Then the disease begins with weariness and depression. A fever, moderate at first increases from day to day, generally attains a considerable height at the end of a week and fourteen days later generally abates. Towards the end of the fourth week in the normal course the fever, and with it the disease proper is usually over; but the patient still requires a long time, after a period of several months, before he attains complete restoration to health. Concomitant and subsequent diseases, such as inflammation of the lungs, suppuration of the skin and joints, pains in the ear, nervous disorders, even mental diseases are frequently associated with typhoid and cause death or the development of infirmities and debility. The disease itself may endanger life, e. g. by exhausting hæmorrhage from the bowels.

The most noteworthy changes produced in the human body by an attack of typhoid consists in the formation of ulcers on the mucous membrane of the small intestines. Moreover swelling of the spleen is always present and besides a more or less pronounced delirium, catarrhs of the respiratory and digestive passages, especially diarrhœa usually complete the form of the disease. Its name of *"nervous fever"*, which is still frequently used, the disease owes to its nervous symptoms.

Patients suffering from typhoid should not fail to obtain *medical treatment*. Where regular visits from a physician are not possible, or where domestic and business conditions make nursing difficult, the patient should certainly be brought into a hospital, where nursing is brought to perfection.

II. Infectious diseases.

In *nursing typhoid patients* special care should be taken that they do not receive solid food before the physician allows it. Compliance caused by false pity with the craving of the patient, tormented by a feeling of hunger during convalescence has often been severely punished, as such diet, being difficult of digestion has led to evil results, even to rupture of the peritoneum, which at the ulcerated spots during healing is reduced to the thinness of paper. Thus the frequently observed relapses of the disease are often connected with the non-observance of the directions, given as to the diet of the patients.

The typhoid germs leave the body of the patient along with the excreta and urine, and easily pass even with careful watching to his linen and bedding; especially as the excretions sometimes occur involuntarily. From his linen the infection germs may pass to his hands and next to all objects, touched by him, such as clothes, food, utensils, and may thus carry infection to relatives, nurses, physicians and other persons, who do not carefully observe the regulations, necessary in the intercourse with the patient. The patient's linen must be disinfected as soon as possible after use, and the sick-room and its furniture after the close of the illness.

The excreta of the patient should never be discharged or removed without previous disinfection. The non-observance of the latter regulation is a frequent cause of epidemics of typhoid, and in fact those houses and houses are especially afflicted with this disease, where the removal of the refuse and the water supply do not comply with sanitary requirements. Where unobjectionable water is not attainable, it is advisable at the outbreak of the disease already to boil all water used, but in any case to drink only boiled water.

§ 203. Gastric fever. Catarrh of the stomach and intestines. Diarrhoea. Unfortunately, the execution of the preventive measures just described is omitted in many cases of typhoid, partly from ignorance or neglect, partly because the disease, on account of its mild symptoms at first is not described as typhoid, but as gastric fever. By this latter term is understood a feverish stomach catarrh, which is produced by unhealthy, putrid or excessive food, and exhibits itself by loss of appetit constipation, headache, pain or feeling of oppression in the abdomen, foul smell from the mouth, hiccough, nausea and vomiting. Typhoid is also sometimes mistaken for intestinal catarrh, which arises from similar causes as gastric catarrh and is characterized by diarrhœa.

The disordered conditions of the digestive organs just mentioned may also appear in an apparently mild form and without fever, but may nevertheless take a serious turn and lead to injurious consequences, especially by injudicious conduct of the patient. It is therefore advisable to call in a physician in such indispositions, and even before his arrival to make the choice of food conformable to the principles indicated further on (cf. § 249).

By simultaneous disorder of the stomach and the intestines *diarrhœa* is produced from similar causes as the last mentioned illness. It often runs its course in the form of a slight indisposition without leaving behind any after-effects, but sometimes it appears as an illness, dangerous to life and then it is called *cholera nostras*. Complaints of this kind are particularly observed in large numbers among children of tender age in summer, particularly in towns (cf. § 157) causing many deaths among small children.

A cause, acting simultaneously on several persons, e. g. the partaking of putrid food (*poisoning by sausages*, cf. also §§ 84, 88, 89) leads sometimes to the falling ill of "a group" of persons from diarrhœa or cholera nostra; but this disease lacks the peculiarity of spreading from the sick to the healthy by the immediate or mediate transmission of infection. It is thus distinguished from one of the most terrible and most dreaded epidemics, with whose course cases of severe diarrhœa possess much similarity, namely asiatic cholera.

§ 204. **Cholera.** *Asiatic cholera*, which has long been indigenous to Asia, especially to India, did not make its appearance in Europe till the 19th century, when it either made its way as a migratory epidemic through Persia to Russia and the Balcan countries, or was imported by seafaring people to the seaports. It then produced epidemics in many European countries, which disappeared after a few years only to break out again upon renewed importation. As an instance of the extent of the devastations, caused by this epidemic, it may be mentioned, that the cholera epidemic of 1892 in the Russian Empire caused 550 000 cases of illness and 260 000 deaths, and in the small territory of the (free seaport) state of

Hamburg caused in a few weeks 18000 cases of illness and 8000 deaths.

The course of a severe case of cholera is somewhat the following: The disease appears with violent vomiting and diarrhœa several hours, but as a rule some days after the reception of the cholera germs. The excretions, becoming more frequent, soon acquire a colourless appearance, similar to thin flour gruel or the water, poured off boiled rice and thus withdraw such considerable quantities of fluid from the body, that the secretion of urine ceases; the skin becomes dried and can be raised in large folds, which only slowly return to their normal level. At the same time severe muscular cramps set in, especially in the calves of the legs; exhaustion rapidly increasing, the patient becomes quite apathic for everything that happens with or around him, and often after a few hours only death already follows.

In less severe cases vomiting ceases after some hours, the excretions become gradually less frequent, resume their normal character and after two or three weeks full convalescence ensues. Patients, who survive the attack of cholera proper frequently succumb to the so-called cholera typhoid, a feverish condition with delirium, which frequently develops at the end of the original disease.

For the purpose of studying this epidemic an Imperial commission of savants, consisting of three members was sent by the German Empire to Egypt and India. R. Koch, as head of this commission of experts succeeded in discovering the germ of the cholera in the form of the comma bacillus, so well known since that time. This bacillus propagates under favourable conditions with uncommon rapidity and spreads in the same manner, as the typhoid germ, especially according to our experience by the means of water, used for domestic purposes or for drinking.

To prevent the spread of the disease the isolation and the disinfection must be carried out far more strictly than in the case of typhoid. In particular, besides the excretions of the patient those of all persons in his vicinity, who are already possibly infected, must be made innocuous. For experience shows, that the infection of cholera can be communicated to others in a severe form by such persons, even though they themselves are not affected. The regulations, mentioned in

§ 153 for the supervision of traffic have proved efficacious in the case of cholera. Especially the establishment of medical stations on the water-ways for the supervision of the *seafaring population* has proved successful and efficient. This precaution was also acknowledged as useful by some foreign states, and was recommended for general adoption at the Congress, held in Dresden by many European Powers in the year 1893 for the purpose of combating the cholera. The success of all precautions will be the more certain; the greater the care taken will be in every household, in every village and town with regard to cleanliness, proper removal of refuse and of the supply of wholesome, pure drinking-water.

During cholera epidemics one should live the usual regular mode of life, avoid medicines, as long as we are healthy, and should not abandon our homes from fear of the disease. Where reliable drinking water cannot be procured, only boiled water should be used for domestic purposes as well as for drinking. We should avoid eating ice, very cold beverages, bad beer, unboiled milk, and such food or drinks or luxuries or refreshments, which might cause disorders in our digestion. We should obtain our provisions and food only from reliable, clean shops and should avoid to get those things from shops in houses where a case of cholera occurred. We should not bathe in rivers or lakes, near which cases of cholera occurred, and use public privies only in case of urgent need. The seats of privies used by strangers should be scrubbed daily with soap and water. Those, used by persons, suspected of cholera, should be sprinkled with chloride of lime. If our digestion is in the least degree out of order, one should see at once a physician.

§ 205. **Dysentery.** *Dysentery* belongs to the diseases of an epidemic character, arising from morbid changes in the intestines. It is a widely extended disease in southern countries, but has also caused sometimes epidemics in our country; in some parts of Germany it appears regularly at certain seasons. In cases of dysentery the patient suffers from inflammation and ulcers in the great intestine especially in the rectum. The patient has high fever and is continually tortured by efforts to relieve his bowels. The frequent excretions, always painful are mixed with mucous, pus, and blood. In favourable cases reconvalescence gradually sets in after 2 or

3 weeks, frequently the disease lasts a longer time; severe attacks sometimes cause death. The infectious matter of dysentery so far, as is known is disseminated by the excretions of the patients; as a safeguard against its spreading the precautions as against typhoid should be employed.

§ 206. **Diphtheria, Croup, Tonsillitis.** An infectious disease, dreaded in childhood, but also affecting adults, is *diphtheria*. The number of deaths, caused by it among the ten million inhabitants of the larger towns in Germany during the ten years 1882—1891 amounted to 111,021 and of every thousand deaths 45 are due to this disease. In 1892 the death-rate from diphtheria was 12361, or 41 per 1000.

The disease usually begins with fever and pains in the throat; on the inflamed and swollen tonsils appear grayish-white dots, which soon increase to a uniform coating, and generally cover also the uvula and the upper part of the throat. At the same time the lymphatic glands in the neek become swollen, the breath of the patient is foul, and the nose becomes obstructed. Often death ensues in a few days; either from failure of the heart's action, or from swelling of the mucous membrane of the larynx and windpipe, rendering breathing impossible. In other cases, after diseases, such as inflammation of the lungs or kidneys and paralysis, produce a fatal result or tedious recovery. In consequence of laryngeal muscles paralysis, hoarseness and loss of voice may remain after the disease has passed away.

A formation of a membranous coating inside the larynx and branches of the windpipe sometimes occurs without a previous affection of the throat; such cases result in a peculiar form of disease, distinguished by want of breath and symptoms of choking and called "croup". Such a condition of things is called "true croup", as opposed to "false croup" a catarrhal disease of the air passages, which is accompanied by swelling of the mucous membrane, want of breath and danger of suffocation, but not by the formation of a membrane.

Every attack of diphtheria threatens the life of the person attacked; prompt and proper treatment may obtain successful results.[1]) A physician may succeed in averting the imminent

---

[1]) It is therefore advisable to look into the throat af a child, as soon as it complains of being ill.

danger of suffocation as soon as "*croup*" appears, by making *the incision in the trachea*, below the larynx obstructed by the membranous coating and thus providing a free passage of air to the lungs. But the patient's life is not always saved by this operation, for by preventing suffocation only one of the manifold dangers, occasioned by diphtheria is removed. As absolutely efficient can be recommended the use of the diphtheria serum, introduced by v. Behring in 1894 called "Diphtheria healing sérum"; this is obtained from the serum of the blood of horses, which has acquired a high capacity for resisting the disease owing to repeated inoculations with the diphtheria poison (cf. § 189). How great the decrease of mortality in diphtheria during recent years was, the following figures will show: In the ten German states, which since 1892 have taken part in the common statistics of the causes of deaths there died, in the years 1892—1898 of this disease 55746, 75322, 63162, 37527, 31503, 25788 and 23642 persons; i. e. for every 100000 inhabitants 118.8, 158.2, 130.9, 76.5, 64.2, 51.7 and 46.9. In Prussia these numbers were 130.2, 177.6, 144.9, 88.1, 74.6, 60.7 and 54.8. In Bavaria 86.3, 100.0, 84.5, 47.6, 39.4, 31.4, 33.7; in Saxony 105.0, 106.2, 93.4, 69.4, 57.2, 40.6 and 36; in Wurtemberg 178.5, 218.0, 196.7, 85.4, 61.7, 45.1 and 47.2. Already in the year 1894, (but still more considerable in 1895, when the diphtheria-healing-serum came into more general use) a decrease in the mortality from diphtheria to $\frac{1}{3}$ and $\frac{1}{4}$ of the previous year's numbers is shown. The alleged efficacy of a great number of special healing remedies, which are "praised up" every year by various means on the part of non-medical persons; especially the efficiency of "secret remedies" (cf. § 145) has never been proved; especially in serious cases of diphtheria these remedies had no effect, and they cannot be recommended by medical science. The testimonials, given to the dealers in such remedies are generally based upon the mistake of considering as diphtheria milder diseases of a similar order, e. g. the different forms of *tonsillitis*.

This disease frequently appears together with high fever and a very noticeable swelling of the dark-red tonsils, and next a whitish coating, similar to the coating in diphtheria may show itself. Sometimes there appears a collection of matter inside the tonsils, which, unless an incision is quickly made, gradually bursts into the mouth, causing great pain to the patient. Apart from a few rare exceptional cases tonsillitis usually ends favourably in a few days, without leaving any after-diseases.

According to our experience it is not impossible that tonsillitis may also be transmitted from one person to another. But *diphtheria* is the more dangerous *contagious* disease. Its germs adhere particularly to the lining of the throat, pass thence into the saliva of the patient, also into the discharges from the nose and seem to remain for a long time capable of transferring infection with dried expectoration in dwelling-rooms, linen, clothing and utensils.

To prevent the spreading of diphtheria the precautions, used in scarlatina are to be recommended; special care should be taken to render the expectorations of diphtheria patients especially their pocket-handkerchiefs harmless by immersing them immediately after use in disinfecting fluids. Kissing persons, afflicted with diphtheria should be rigorously forbitten and absolutely avoided.

§ 207. **Whooping-cough.** This infectious disease *whooping-cough*, or (*choking cough*, commonly called) is almost exclusively confined to children under ten years of age. The disease begins with the symptoms of a common, ordinary catarrh in the windpipe; perhaps after a week prolonged and violent fits of coughing set in, during which the child gets "blue" in the face and seems to be choking. Each fit usually ends with a deep whistling inspiration whence the disease has received its name, "whooping-cough". Only a little phlegm is usually expectorated by the coughing, yet the violent irritation often causes vomiting. The attacks, which deprive especially at night frequently the sleep of the children, become less frequent and violent after some time, and finally cease altogether. In unfavourable cases, especially with weak children death sometimes ensues from exhaustion, or as a result of inflammation of the lungs.

The infectious matter of whooping cough, it is thought, adheres to the phlegm, expectorated, when coughing, which is frequently very small in quantity. The disease is easily communicated, either directly by the intercourse of healthy children with those affected, or by means of pocket-handkerchiefs. Children, suffering from whooping cough should be always isolated and especially should not be allowed to attend schools. Their linen is disinfected in the simplest way by thorough boiling.

§ 208. Influenza. Like whooping-cough, *Influenza* or *"grippe"* favours most frequently the respiratory organs as the seat of its manifestation. Influenza has repeatedly crossed Europe in its wanderings and has then attacked the majority of the inhabitants of the country, afflicted by it. The beginning of the last great epidemic was in 1889. For explaining the spread of the disease there are not wanting many observations of a communication of the virus from person to person; still a great influence in the promotion of the spread of the disease must be found in the conditions of the weather and of a great many other circumstances.

"Grippe" appears with more or less high fever, with great debility of the patient, painful twinges in the limbs and violent headache. As a rule coughing with expectorations sets in, and in other cases stomach and intestinal catarrh. Recovery usually begins after a few days; still a continuance of weakness and sometimes even death takes place. Inflammation of the lungs, diseases of the heart, ear and kidneys; concomitant and consequential diseases of the "grippe" are the cause of such unfavourable results.

§ 209. Inflammation of the lungs. Pleurisy. Peritonitis. The inflammation of the lungs, appearing both as an independent malady and also in conjunction with other infectious diseases varies greatly in symptoms, course and results, according to its cause.

In the term "inflammation of the lungs" we include various morbid processes, usually accompanied by fever, which, in consequence of a filling up of the lung vesicles with secretions, cause sometimes small and sometimes large portions of the lungs to become incapable of taking part in the function of respiration. The patients are thus obliged to hasten their respiration (want of breath) and suffer pain in the affected parts of the lungs.

The illness usually called "inflammation of the lungs" usually begins with a violent shivering frost and is marked by high fever, stitches in the sides and want of breath. Together with a painful cough, the patients expectorate first only scanty, but afterwards large quantities of viscous phlegm, coloured like iron rust from an admixture of blood. If the patient takes proper care of himself, inflammation of the lungs has a favourable issue more frequently, than might be thought considering the severity of the symptoms. About a week after its commencement the fever and want of breath generally suddenly cease and convalescence follows together while the pain in the chest and the want of breath cease. If the disease runs this course, the secretions in the lung are either coughed up, or absorbed by the lymph-vessels. In serious cases perilous suppuration and other destructive disorders of the lungs may occur. Sometimes death ensues-after a few days already, especially in the case of weakly aged persons or those, weakened by excessive indulgence in alcohol.

Inflammation of the lungs was formerly numbered among diseases, brought on by a cold, but lately we began to consider it as an infectious disease, the origin of which is apparently favoured by influences of the weather; yet is connected with living micro-organisms.

On the supposition, that the latter are disseminated by the dried and dust-blown expectoration of the patient, it is advisable to disinfect all such expectoration and the handkerchiefs, linen etc.

Sometimes the *disease of pleurisy* follows after an inflammation of the lungs. Pleurisy is a disease, endangering the life of the patient, which frequently develops independently; it causes secretion of the fluid in the space between the lungs and the pleura, and often in such large quantities, that breathing becomes difficult or impossible through interference with the movements of the lungs. In some cases the secretion shows a bloody or purulent character.

In *peritonitis* or *inflammation of the abdomen*, which sometimes follows injuries to, or other diseases in the covering of the abdomen or abdominal organs, a watery or purulent fluid is secreted by the peritoneum. The patients usually suffer violent pains and frequently succumb to this dangerous disease.

§ 210. Epidemic stiff-neck. Inflammation of the cerebral membrane.

By the term *epidemic stiff neck* is characterized a feverish infectious disease, which is caused by inflammation of the membranes, surrounding the brain and spinal chord, and in its course is accompanied by vomiting, violent pains in the head, neck and limbs, stiffness of the neck, and paralysis of individual muscles. The disease sometimes spreads widely, especially in winter and spring, amongst children and young persons and ends fatally in about one third of the cases. In cases of recovery, deafness, blindness maiming and mental disorder often remain behind.

Similar to the stiff-neck inflammation of the cerebral membrane makes its appearance. This disease is especially dreaded as an after disease of several infectious diseases, as well as in connection with injuries to the head and diseases of the ear.

§ 211. **Intermittent fever.** A disease, which also owes its origin to micro-organisms is *intermittent fever* or cold fever (malaria). This disease is communicated by special kinds of mosquitoes to man, in whose body these *malaria* parasites pass a part of their development. Intermittent fever occurs especially in marshy districts, often exposed to inundations, and is indigenous in some parts of Germany; but in our climate this disease as a rule is not fatal to human life. In hot climates this *"fever"* (as it is generally called) appears much more frequently and under very severe forms as virulent malarial or tropical fever.

The cases of this disease, observed in our climate are characterized by attacks of high fever, lasting for several hours, recurring every three or four days and usually introduced by shivering; the health of the person attacked is lowered even during the intervals, free from fever. Instead of attacks of fever, violent pains of the nerves (especially in the forehead) also interrupted by intervals, may set in. By proper administration of quinine, a medicine obtained from the bark of the cinchona tree, found in South America, our doctors are almost in every case successful in combating the diseases and see the patient recover his health. By the draining of swamps, regulation of river-beds etc. one very frequently succeeds to banish this disease from districts, formerly ravaged by it.

§ 212. **The Plague.** The *plague*, also called oriental bubonic plague has its home outside of our Continent, in the interior of Asia and Africa. It has spread lately again from China, and many victims succumbed especially during recent times in Eastern India. Latterly this disease appeared in the most remote and in various parts of the world and made its appearance likewise in different places in Europe. In past centuries it has visited Europe with severe epidemics, and in particular the "black death", an epidemic most probably identical with the present-day plague was the most terrible scourge of the human race. The pestilence is characterized by high fever, delirium and swelling of the lymphatic glands on the neck, in the armpits and groin (glandial-plague); in some cases the pestilence appears with symptoms of a severe inflammation of the lungs (lung-plague). The swollen glands assume the form of red protuberances, become festering and burst-gangrenous. The majority of persons attacked die within the first week.

The plague can be communicated directly from an infected person, as well as by means of infected clothes and other objects to healthy persons. The lung-plague is justly dreaded as the most infectious pestilence. Sometimes the infectious matter adheres tenaciously to certain dwellings and houses.

Besides human beings certain animals are particularly apt to spread the infection by means of the plague bacillus; among these animals are to be specially mentioned the rodents and particularly rats. They have great importance in spreading this pestilence.

We combat this terrible epidemic by strict separation of all sick persons and those persons under suspicion of being infected; as well as by the most thorough disinfecting of all objects, which came into contact with a person attacked by the plague. The collection of any kind of refuse within, or in the neighbourhood of human dwellings and the destruction of all rats belongs to the most necessary measures of precaution, as the pestilence caused the most terrible ravages in places that are not kept scrupulously clean.

§ 213. Yellow fever.

The *yellow fever*, a most dangerous disease occurs particularly in the countries near the coast of Central and South America. The increased speed of sea going vessels seems however to justify the fear, that the infectious matter may occasionally also find entrance and propagation in German seaports. The illness is characterized by high fever, headache and pains in the back, a yellow colour of the skin and eybrows (conjunctiva) vomiting of bloody matter, anxiety and talking wildly and the malady usually runs its course in 10—12 days, unless death ensues before. Recovery usually takes a long time.

It is assumed, that yellow fever can be communicated by person to person as well, as by means of clothes and other objects.

§ 214. Wound diseases.

A series of infectious diseases are designated as wound diseases, because their origin is associated with the presence of abrasions in the skin; their excitants are found in dust, dirt or impure water. We can prevent the entrance of disease germs by avoiding as much as possible to touch the wounds, by cleansing scrupulously the edges of the wounds and by using as bandages only *aseptic* (free from putridity germs) bandage material, e. g. cotton-wool gauze etc. We should not omit, before putting on a bandage, cleaning the hands for several minutes with soap and a brush, and removing the dirt from under the nails. The material for bandages should be obtained only from a very reliable source (a chemist's shop) should be taken out from a fresh package every time, and the bandage laid upon the wound with that part, which was not touched by the hand. After use the bandage material should be burnt; in no case should it be used again. The carrying out of these precautions as well as bandaging itself cannot be learned without much practice, and therefore the treatment of wounds should be left to trained hands only, if possible. Wound diseases were formerly very frequent. Pain from inflammation and fever were considered as pain from the wound and fever was considered as a regular and necessary concomitant of the healing process; it was considered unavoidable, that several and even severe wound diseases should appear epidemically among the wounded in lazarettos (military hospitals). Not before the introduction of the so-called "*anti-septic*" (preventing putridity) treatment of wounds by the English physician (now Lord) Lister, in which the highest importance is attached to cleanliness in dealing with wounds, these diseases were observed in exceptional cases only.

§ 215. **Inflammation; Suppuration; Whitlow furuncle, Carbuncle.** The most frequent wound disease is a simple inflammation of the tender parts near the wound; its characteristics are painfulness, swelling redness, heat and fever; sometimes *formation* of *matter* may be added to these symptoms.

This matter gathers particularly in the tissues of the underskin, destroys the latter partially and can acquire considerable dimensious especially in the case of superficial abrasions, which have remained unobserved, until it breaks through the opposing cutticle and is discharged externally. A timely incision may limit in such cases the extent and duration of a *suppuration*.

By the name of *whitlow, worm* or *panaritium* we designate an inflammation, generall caused by small unnoticed abrasions, usually on the inside of the finger, which may lead easily to suppuration; but, if neglected it may lead to more serious consequences, such as destruction of the sinews, stiffening of the finger or of the wrist or even of the arm, incapacitating even the latter; nay by spreading to other parts of the body it may even endanger life. One should not delay in such cases to call in promptly a physician.

A confined collection of matter is called an *abscess* or *purulent boil.* A circumscribed inflammation of the skin, whose origin is often untraceable, and is to be sought in a skin gland, that has become accessible to one of the excitants of inflammation is known as a *boil* or *furuncle.* If several boils lie close to each other, they unite in a carbuncle, which sometimes becomes dangerous to life.

§ 216. **Inflammation of the lymph vessels. Inflammation of the lymph glands. Purulent and putrid fever. Puerperal fever.** If the disease germs, present in the wound, or in the inflamed portions of the skin pass into the lymph vessels, *inflammation of these vessels* or *glands* arise. The vessels become visible as painful red cords, noticeable through the skin and running to the lymph-glands·lying nearest the wound. The latter will become painful and may finally suppurate. If certain inflammatory agents pass through the sides of the small veins into the blood, and by the latter into the other organs, the serious diseases, known as *purulent* or *putrid* fever may appear. *Puerperal fever* an illness of women in childbed sometimes also takes the form of the above mentioned diseases. The puerperal fever arises from the penetration of inflammatory agents into the parts, injured in delivery. Like every wound disease, puerperal fever can only be avoided by great care and scrupulous observance of all regulation concerning cleanlines on the parts of the persons, assisting at the confinement.

§ 217. **Erysipelas and gangrene.** *Erysipelas* appears first in the neighbourhood of wounds as a painful inflammation of the skin, distinguised by swelling and a certain rosy-red colouring. It soon spreads further and may sometimes, as migratory erysipelas, cover a great portion of the surface of the body. It commences with shivering, runs its course, accompanied by high fever, and therefore gives the impression of a grave illness. Erysipelas in the head and face, which were formerly classed among the illnesses arising from a cold, is a wound disease, whose starting point is minute abrasions, e. g. small spots of the mucous membranes, that have become injured from catarrh. Relatively seldom does erysipelas end fatally; most illnesses, caused by it run a favourable course, as the fever ceases after about a weeks duration, and the cuticle scales on the parts affected, the hair usually falls out, but soon grows again.

A local dying off of portions of the body sometimes occuring after wounds is known as gangrene. Frequently it develops into complete destruction of the parts near the wound, and often causes the total loss of limbs, and even the death of the person attacked. Its name is derived from the dark almost black colour of the parts affected. Similar appearances are observed on other occasions, e. g. frost-bites (§ 183), or even independently in consequence of obstructed circulation (gangrene senilis).

§ 218. **Tetanus.** *Tetanus*, on account of its almost certain issue, and of the tortures, endured by the patient is one of the most dreaded wound diseases. Opening of the mouth, chewing, swallowing breathing become difficult, owing to painful spasms of the jaw, neck and larynx. The spasms subsequently disappear, but the slightest contact, emotions, even auditory and visual sensations may recall them with lightning speed. Similar spasms extend to the entire body, repeat themselves constantly, thereby enfeebling the body and exhausting its strength to such a degree, that few patients survive their sufferings.

§ 219. **Contagious diseases of the eye.** *Inflammations of the tunics of the eyes* arise like wound diseases from the entrance of dirt or dust. The mucous membrane becomes red, effusion of tears increase with the secretion of matter, pains in the eye and·avoidance of light ensue. Occasionally there are formed on the edges of the eyelids swellings resembling boils, called „sties". If the inflammation passes from the conjunctiva, the outer covering, to the cornea, ulcers are produced on the latter, which leave behind scars, impeding the power of vision, these scars are called *spots on the cornea*. A simultaneous affection of the inner parts of the eye may occasion diminution of the visual power, blindness and loss of the eye.

II. Infectious diseases.

One of the most dangerous forms of inflammation of the conjunctiva, the infections *eye-disease of new-born children* has been already mentioned. (§ 158.) Another infectious form, the *contagious or infectious eye-disease* also called *trachoma* is a very extensively spread disease, which has been known in Egypt since the very remotest ages. There at the end of the eighteenth century Napoleon's soldiers were attacked by it. In Europe the disease has been prevalent for many centuries. It still makes its appearance sometimes in some parts of Germany by the name of the *Egyptian* or *granular* eye-disease. The communication of this very dangerous eye-disease is effected by means of the hands, towels etc. We should therefore be on our guard against contact with patients suffering from this disease and should never use their linen without previous disinfection. The spread of the disease is most reliably prevented by submitting immediately to proper treatment as soon as attacked.

§ 220. Contagious animal diseases. Certain *infectious diseases of animals* are sometimes communicated to men as wound-diseases, if their germs find admission into the human body by means of existing abrasions or through bites. Such diseases of animals are hydrophobia, anthrax and glanders.

§ 221. Hydrophobia. Rabies, or hydrophobia is a disease, most frequently observed in dogs; its virus is contained in the saliva of the animals affected, and is transferred to human beings by the animal licking sore parts of the skin or by bites. Such transfers result in a great many cases in a severe illnes of the person affected, the outbreak of which usually takes place after a period of between twenty to sixty days; sometimes even later after the infection. The patients first experience weariness, headache, pain and difficulty in speaking or swallowing. After a few days or hours cramp ensues in the muscles used in swallowing and breathing, especially in making an effort to drink, and subsequently even at the thought of drinking or swallowing. These attacks may also take place on other trifling irritations, such as draughts, looking at shining objects, sudden contact etc. Their frequent repetition causes a rapidly — increasing weakness, and leads in a few days to the death of the patient. To prevent the development of the disease it is considered useful to suck, cut, burn or cauterize wounds, caused by the bite of suspicious animals. In France and other countries, where rabies occurs far more frequently than in Germany, institutes for inoculation against rabies have been established at the instigation of the famous analytical chemist Pasteur; a similar institute exists in Berlin since 1898 in connection with the institute for infectious diseases. The sooner the bitten persons are sent to these institutes, the more certain is their cure.

§ 222. Anthrax. Glanders.

Anthrax attacks particularly sheep and cattle; more seldom pigs and horses. It is produced by a rod-like bacillus, which is contained in large numbers in the blood and in many organs of the diseased animals, and can also be artificially reared outside their bodies without losing its activity. As the anthrax bacilles forms spores, the infectious matter of the disease may retain its power and capacity of transmitting virus for a long time, e. g. in coagulated blood. Its transfer to men may be effected by means of the flesh, horns or skin; the slaughtering and skinning of the animals, and the working up of their hides and hair offer thereto the occasion. The virus may also, as it seems, be introduced into the human body by the bite of insects, that have been sitting upon the diseased animals.

In man the disease shows itself generally by the so-called anthrax carbuncle, a circumscribed and very violent inflammation of the skin, accompanied by pustules and burning sensations, or it appears as the more extensive anthrax swelling, but marked in its course by the same symptoms. By the passage of diseased substances from the original seat into the track of the blood a dangerous general sickness may be produced along with high fever. Diseases arising from the eating of the flesh of animals, afflicted with anthrax, and characterized at first by violent vomiting and diarrhœa run a similar course.

Glanders appear in *horses* and other *one-hoofed animals* and may be communicated to man by the mucus from the animals nose, the secretion of skin ulcers, by the blood, by the sweat, saliva, urine and milk of such animals; it is most frequently transferred by the virus, penetrating skin wounds. Ulcers and inflammations of the lymph-vessels and neighbouring lymph-glands are produced at the point of entry of the disease germs. This is followed by fever, pains in the limbs, pustular skin eruptions and the production of deeply-seated tubercles which break and form ulcers. Even in the nose and in the inner parts of the body tubercles may develop and other inflammatory changes. The disease almost without exception results in death in a short time or after periods, extending over months, sometimes even years. By burning or cauterizing the wounds or ulcers, suspected of being infected the disease may sometimes be prevented.

§ 223. Other diseases of animals, which may be communicated to man.

Among other animals diseases various skin diseases (*scab* in horses and dogs, *ringworm*) caused by various animal and vegetable parasites may spread to man; this is also the case with the foot and mouth disease, noticed particularly among cattle, sheep and pigs. The virus of the latter is found particularly in small pustules in the mouth, in the neighbourhood of the feet and on the udder of diseased animals and may be communicated through the use of unboiled milk, or by soiling the hands and the face in tending animals. The diseases, caused by *trichinae*, *fins* and other parasites transferred sometimes to man by eating animal flesh have been already mentioned (§ 83). The serious danger to health, which may be caused by the dog tape-worm will be noticed later or (§ 231).

§ 224. Syphilis. This illness is caused almost exclusively by direct contact with the infected persons; it is unfortunately a very widely spread malady, which at first is characterized frequently in very insignificant looking ulcers only or in swellings of the glands and skin-eruptions; but which during its course affects various organs; e. g. the bones, brain and the spinal cord, and may lead to a complete derangement of the body. Frequently it is inherited by children from their parents. Patients are urgently advised, to see a physician as quickly as possible.

§ 225. Leprosy.

Lepra causes prolonged and serious chronic illness. This disease, which is also infectious, is widely spread throughout the Orient, but it also still makes its appearance in other countries, especially in some parts of Europe, as for instance in Norway, some provinces of Russia, Turkey and Spain. In Germany, where at present there are only very few lepers, their number in former years was so considerable, that every large town had its special leper hospital for such patients ("leproserien").

The disease is characterized by the devolopment of tubercles and eruptions on the skin and by nervous-disorders; but in its course it also attacks other organs and after lasting for several years leads to death. In places, visited by this disease they try to protect the healthy by isolating those who are afflicted with leprosy from all intercourse with others.

§ 226. Tuberculosis. A number of externally very dissimilar diseases, all of which almost are *chronic*, are included under the name of *tuberculosis*. The proof, that these apparently dissimilar maladies have a common origin, and therefore are essentially of the same nature, has been brought a few years ago by Professor Koch's discovery of the tubercle bacillus. This micro-organism, which is found in all diseases, connected with tuberculosis, which can also remain infectious outside the human body and also may even propagate outside the body, causes within the body the formation of small tubercles and the production of inflammatory processes. Decay, destruction and ulceration ensue, because the tubercles and the inflamed tissue gradually change into a dry, white, crumbling mass, resembling cheese, with concomitant suppuration. The ulcers form the entrance-gate for other disease germs, by whose agency the characteristic symptoms of the disease may be changed in various ways.

A frequent co-symptom of tuberculosis is the so-called *hectic fever*, which causes considerable rises in the temperature of the body at definite periods of the day, especially in the evening, and together with profuse perspiration at night weakens the patient. Sometimes this fever betrays itself in the patient at an early stage already by sharp-edged red spots on the cheeks, which become specially visible during slight exertion, sense impressions and emotions.

§ 227. **Individual forms of tuberculosis.** The most frequent form of tuberculosis is *pulmonary consumption*. Between 1886 and 1895 it carried off yearly on the average about 33,963 persons of the twelve millions urban inhabitants in Germany, i. e. about three in every thousand, and it caused about 12 percent of all deaths. Its outward characteristics are, besides the general symptoms of tuberculosis, especially coughing, expectorating and want of breath. Frequently bleeding occurs as a result of the destruction of the sides of the lung vesicles and shows itself in a bloody colour of the expectoration (*blood-spitting*, *blood-coughing*); sometimes it increases to a dangerous extent, and may lead to throwing up considerable quantities of blood (*violent haemorrhage of the lungs*).

Tuberculosis sometimes appears in the bones, resulting in *caries*, i. e. extensive *destruction of the bones*. If the dorsal vertebræ are the starting point of such a disease, there is formed a projecting knob on the back, corresponding to the seat of the disease by the sinking in of the decaying vertebral body. At the same time may arise injury or concomitant disease of the spinal chord, and in consequence thereof, paralysis of the lower limbs, or difficulty in the urinary organs and bowels. Tubercular disease of the ends of the bones may easily extend into the *neighbouring joints*. The former at first causes pains and limping and in its further stages it may lead to suppuration, destruction of the joint, loss of the limb (voluntary limping), and even death.

The tuberculosis of the cerebral membranes especially frequent in the case of very young children is marked at first by depression and digestive troubles; soon however loss of consciousness, convulsions and paralysis appear, and almost without exception the disease ends fatally in a few weeks. Still more quickly destroying is *general Tuberculosis* (acute miliar), which arises, when the bacilli from a local seat of the disease spread suddenly throughout the whole body. Fever, similar to typhoid appears and the disease ends fatally in a very few weeks. Tuberculosis in the intestines, mesentery and abdomen quickly puts an end to life.

Among the tuberculous skin diseases *lupus* must be mentioned, a disease which especially appears in the face, destroys and disfigures it sometimes entailing the entire loss of the nose.

§ 228. **Scrofula. Curable nature of tuberculosis.** Under the general term of *scrofulosis* (scrofulous diseases) we characterize some tedious skin diseases arising from tuberculosis and also the tubercular gland maladies, characterized by swelling, whitening, suppuration and ulceration; it is accompanied sometimes by an inflammation of the cornea, marked by a slow course and a tendency to relapses; and also with manyfold maladies of the ear, accompanied by suppuration. Formerly it was thought, that these maladies and also the above mentioned affection of the bones are quite different diseases, and not tuberculosis, because they occur almost always in the case of children, and have generally a more favourable termination than the above mentioned tubercular diseases. But with evidence of the bacillus of tuberculosis in the afflicted parts of the body the tuberculous nature of some of these scrofulous diseases was recognized and the former belief in incurability of tuberculosis was at once abandoned. In fact even consumption not unfrequently may end in *recovery*; the cases, which have terminated favourably, have been recognized, when the patients have afterwards died of other diseases and the post-mortem examination has revealed the traces of past lung disease. Cases also, in which pronounced symptoms of tuberculosis are present, can by prompt and proper treatment be cured, or at least receive such a favourable turn, that life and working power are preserved for many years to the patient. There should be no delay therefore to call in a doctor, if persistent coughs, expectoration, mixed with traces of blood decline in bodily weight, digestive troubles, pains in the points etc. raise the suspicion of the presence of tuberculosis.

§ 229. **Dissemination of tuberculosis and preventive measures against it.** Since the discovery of the bacillus of tuberculosis, we have much more reliable information with regard to the manner, in which this *disease* is *disseminated*, we are of course well aware of the fact, that the predisposition to the disease can be transmitted from parents to children, and that a chance cold may prepare the ground for consumption. But at the present time the cause of the propagation of the disease is primarily looked for in the transfer of live disease germs. It is proved that these germs leave the patients's bodies with their excretions, e. g. expectorations, matter, or excreta from the bowels, and retain their vitality even after they dry up. These germs have been found in the dust of bedrooms and other apartments, occupied by tubercular patients, and thus have been traced many cases of tuberculosis, arising from living with such patients or among the dwellers of apartments, which have been occupied by them. Since the *murrain*, a very frequent cattle disease has been recognized as tuberculosis, the conviction has gained ground, that the milk of diseased cows propagates the disease, especially among children.

These observations and the experience gained make it appear urgently advisable to render the excretions of persons, afflicted with consumption quite innocuous, that the danger arising from the intercourse of such persons with healthy persons should be averted as far as possible, and that the use of milk, containing tubercle bacilli should be prohibited. To this end the following regulations may be recommended.[1])

1. All persons, but particularly those, proved to be afflicted by the disease, should accustom themselves to deposit their expectorations in spittoons. These should contain either fluids, which will prevent the expectoration from drying up and turning into dust, or easily combustible substances, such as sawdust. They should be emptied at least once a day, and the contents be made innocuous by burning them or by disinfection. Where the use of spittoons is impossible, as in

---

[1]) Cf. The *Memorandum on tuberculosis*, prepared by the *Imperial Board of Health;* Jul. Springer, Berlin, price 5 pf. and the 'pricecrowned" essay „Tuberculosis as the people's disease" by Dr. S. E. Knopf, physician in New York.

taking a walk in the street, such patients should carry with them vessels (see picture 43) for the contents of their expectorations; but they should never spit on the floor or in their pocket-handkerchiefs.

2. Linen and utensils of the patients should be thoroughly boiled each time after use; their dwellings should be disinfected, before they are occupied by other persons.

3. No dust should be allowed to remain in the dwelling rooms of consumptives. Curtains with many folds, thick carpets and other furniture which absorbs much dust should be replaced by flat objects, easily washed.

4. The sleeping together of consumptives and healthy persons in the same rooms or beds should be avoided as much as possible. Where consumptives and healthy people have to work together, the director of the works should draw their attention to the above measures of caution under 1.

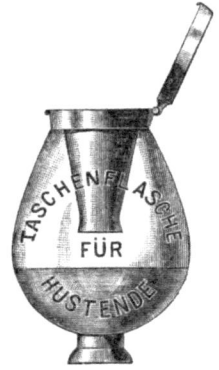

Fig. 43.
Pocket-flask for Coughing.

5. The sale of milk of cows, affected with tuberculosis should be forbidden. The use of unboiled milk is generally to be avoided unless its perfectly reliable source is absolutely established.

III. Other diseases.

§ 230. **Diseases of the nerves and the Brain. Disorders in the formation of blood, and the development of the Body.** The group of *nervous diseases* embraces numerous maladies, some of them only investigated closely in recent years. Their external symptoms, e. g. paralysis, weakness, cramps, pains, loss of sensations, of consciousness, of the capacity of thinking, illusions could frequently be traced to certain changes in the brain, in the spinal column or in the nerves; wettings, severe chills, or preceding infections diseases have been made responsible, with more or less justification as the causes of many nervous maladies. In numerous cases mental overexertion, over-excitement of the senses and feelings; a dissolute life, or indulgence in the consumption of too much alcoholic liquors have preceded the disease. Frequently, especially if a change in the nervous organs cannot be proved, despondency and a want of will-power in the patient must bear the onus of the origin and the unfavourable development of the disease.

A number of nervous maladies may be cured by proper treatment of the patient, conducted by experienced physicians; in others such treatment may succeed to affect favourably the course of the disease and to prolong the life. It is therefore advisable to seek medical advice on the appearance of nervous disorders. This especially in cases, when striking loss of memory, irritability, senseless actions and other symptoms lead us to suppose the beginning of a mental disorder. Frequently the threatening evil may still be averted; in any case prompt knowledge of it may restrain the patient from actions, which might have disastrous consequences for the patient or his family.

Through interference with the formation of blood and development, *chlorosis*, a disease very frequent at present in young girls is characterized. Its development may be counteracted by wholesome care of the body, and nourishment. In particular should girls in their youth and during their years of development frequently take exercise in the open air, avoid much sitting, too much brain work, dancing, parties and similar pleasures, which greatly excite them in an unusual manner, last far into the night and shorten their sleep.

Some diseases, which frequently end fatally whose nature is based on changes in the quality of the blood are the so-called "*Leucomia*" (increase of the white corpuscles) and several kinds of *anaemia* (destruction of the red blood-corpuscles). One form of the latter disease is produced by a very small intestinal worm, the Anchylostomum duodenale, which multiplies exceedingly rapidly in the intestines of the patients. This disease has been observed during the last years in some parts of Germany also, where it was imported from abroad; the persons afflicted are generally bricklayers and earth workers.

A very well-known malady is *diabetes*, a disorder in human health, the origin of which is not yet sufficiently known. In it the urine of the patients, evacuated in considerably increased quantity contains grape sugar. The illness is first marked by an unusually large feeling of hunger and thirst, then by a condition of weariness and weakness; it may lead to death in a few months through improper treatment. But if the patients regulate their lives conscientiously according to the advice, working power and life may be preserved for a long time yet.

Gout is produced by the deposition in various parts of the body of salts, which usually are excreted by the urine. It appears mostly with interruptions in the form of attacks, leads to painful swellings of the points, and prefers among these that between the middle of the foot and the great toe. It also produces "gouty knots" in the skin and diseases of the internal organs. According to popular belief, this malady particularly seeks out those persons, who prefer high living; but it is a fact, that gout is as frequent a malady among the needy and even among persons, exposed to want. By a plain, healthy mode of life the number of attacks may be limited and life prolonged.

§ 231. Tumours and Cancer. Many so-called *tumours* produce a tedious malady and frequently end fatally. By tumours we understand morbid new-structures, which may develop on the surface and in the interior of the body, and possess as a rule a tissue differing in quality from the part of the body affected.

According to their nature we distinguish between *benign and malignant* new-structures. The first named include among others the encysted and fatty; they are distinguished from the malign (the chief members of which are *cancerous*) tumours by their growth being confined to the place, where they first originated, and the absence of a general disease. A benign tumour may cause disfigurement and disorders by its place and size; it may even endanger life by its growth, if its seat is in a vital organ. But it neither produces other secondary tumours in other parts of the body, nor as a rule symptoms of general disease or disorders in nourishment. The removal of a benign growth by an operation destroys immediately and permanently the disorders arising from it. Whereas on the other hand a malignant tumour besides its rapid growth frequently shows the disposition to propagate itself. In the neighbourhood of a cancerous growth there sometimes develop similar tumours of the lymphatic glands, and some time afterwards cancerous knots appear in various parts of the body, remote from the original seat of the disease. At the same time such tumours sometimes break open, decay into ulcers on the surface and discharge matter which generally has a foul smell. The patients suffer pain and other inconveniences, owing to the seat of the tumour, they commence to languish; marasmus sets in and they die, unless the surgeon succeeds to remove the tumour by an operation. Unfortunately in most cases help comes too late, as the danger from the growth, which at first only appears as a small knot, is under-estimated as a rule, and the surgeon's knife is dreaded until the development of more considerable troubles. As soon as the disease has extended further and beyond the lymph glands near the original seat, it is generally no longer possible to avert an unfavourable issue. If in such cases an operation is performed, it is done only for the purpose of alleviating the patient's condition by removing the suppurating ulcers and the troublesome parts of the tumour, and to prolong the patient's life for a short time. The prompt, timely surgical operation at the commencement of the disease is the only means hitherto known to heal cancer; all other recommendations of remedies, which in great numbers proceed sometimes from good intentions, some from love of gain, calculating upon the credulity of the patients only lead to this, that by applying the belauded cures the period for operative treatment is wasted.

A special form of tumours *(echinococcus)* is formed by the *tapeworm of dogs*. This parasite of the dog's intestines, similar in character to the human tapeworm, but only of the thickness of a thread, and hardly over one centimetre long, produces eggs, which pass with the dog's excreta, and are sometimes transferred to human beings by licking. In the intestines of man these eggs grow again to the embryonic form of the worm and in this state pass through the circulation of the blood to the different parts of the body. Here the intruder forms cysts, similar to those in cattle and swine (cf. § 83). These increase in time to larger tumours, which may enclose derivative cysts, and frequently endanger life through being situated in a vital organ, inaccessible to the surgeon, e. g. in the liver or brain. The numerous cases, in which through this disease man languished and even death ensued, urgently caution to be prudent in our relations with dogs. Especially children ought to be prevented from being licked by dogs.

IV. Accidents.

§ 232. Frequency of accidents. Value of the first assistance offered. Various kinds of accidents. Accidents occupy a prominent place among the external influences, injurious to health. During the decade 1886 to 1895 among every 100000 inhabitants of the larger towns of Germany there died in every year 33 in consequence of "*accidents*". The number of temporary or lasting injuries to health, resulting from accidents is to be computed in a much larger number, as for instance in 1892 besides 6000 fatal "accidents" there occurred 49000 other accidents, for which the trades insurance unions had to pay compensation to the injured persons.

The way of preventing accidents was mentioned above (§ 179). The removal or lessening of their consequences does not a little depend on the quickness, with which professional assistance is rendered to the injured. Any loss of time may be prejudicial to the injured; therefore the doctor is not to be waited for in every case, but measures should be taken as soon as possible for the relief of the sufferer. But this can be done only, if the persons present to render the first assistance know the necessary measures to be adopted, and apply their knowledge with prudence. We try therefore to make the information as to first aid to be given in accidents accessible to the widest classes of people, and to spread the knowledge necessary for this purpose by printed instructions as well as by oral teaching in so-called "samaritan schools", in the army, in the civil service and among working men's societies.

To the injuries to health, caused by accident belong the injuries from violence burns and corrodings, poisonings, light and severe case of fainting, the different kinds of so-called "apparent death", and the intrusion of foreign objects into the human body.

At the attempts of rescue all unnecessary visitors should be removed.

§ 233. Wounds and bleedings. Injuries, causing a cutting of the skin are called *wounds*. Their importance depends on their size, their depth, the locality of the injury and the course of the process of healing. Cicatrization ensues most speedily, if (as in many cuts from wounds) the edges of the wound can be brought together; the healing process proceeds much slower in extensive wounds, whose surface has first to be filled up by red flesh corpuscles (in large growths also called "wild flesh", and in contusions, whose more or less injured edges break off gradually from the tissue, which has remained sound. Through wound diseases the healing process may be considerable delayed even in cases of slight wounds (§ 214—218).

Wounds should never be touched with a finger, nor be washed with a sponge; neither should we use the popular remedies for stopping bleeding, e. g. cobwebs or tinder, and such like materials, as they only pollute the wound. The supply of linen and lint in a household, even if it appears to be quite clean, is not as a rule so clean, that the presence of dangerous germs in them is excluded; therefore it should not be used for the purpose of stopping bleeding or bandaging wounds. Coagulated blood should not be removed. But if the wound is soiled by sand or otherwise, in case of medical aid not being quickly on hand, the wound should be carefully syringed with water, which has been boiled and cooled again, or with the *weak* (two percent) *solution* of carbolic water, to be obtained in every chemist's shop. For this purpose a syringe or an irrigator, (§ 248) [which has been cleaned with boiling hot water previously] should be used, but one should avoid to let a strong jet of water to strike the wound.

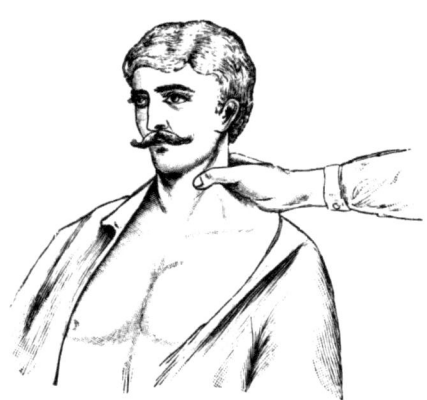

Fig. 44.
Compression of the carotid artery.

Superficial small wounds generally heal quickly when covered with the usual yellow sticking-plaster; larger wounds should be temporarily protected against being soiled by a clean bandage or a handkerchief, fastened by a string, until the surgeon arrives; sometimes however bleeding makes a further quicker treatment desirable.

The nature and danger of bleeding depends on the number and kinds of bloodvessels injured. If the blood trickles from the wound uniformly and not in a strong stream, only the capillary vessels and small veins are injured; a slight pressure by means of a clean bandage fastened by strings on the wound is sufficient to stop the bleeding. A similar, only more firmly attached bandage stops the bleeding from an injured vein, whose character is the welling forth of dark blood in a strong stream (cf. § 16). If the blood spouts in a bright red stream from the wound, or if the blood comes out jerkily, corresponding to the heart's beats, then an artery

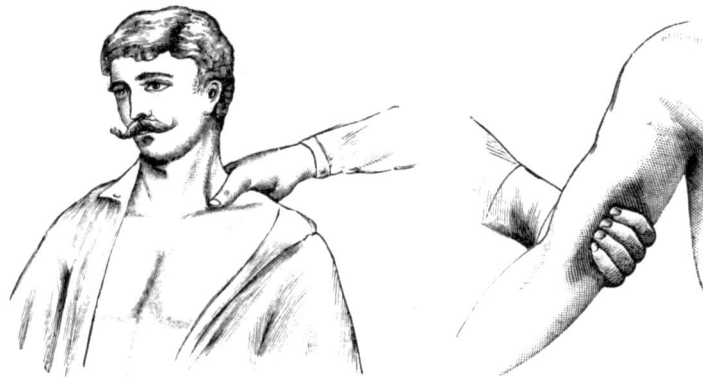

Fig. 45.
Compression of the subclavian artery.

Fig. 46.
Compression of the brachial artery.

has been injured, and a simple bandage is as a rule not sufficient to stop the bleeding, the blood streaming from the open vessel owing to the heart's action. Until the arrival of a surgeon, who is able to find the injured artery in the wound and tie it, the flow of blood may be prevented by pressing the trunk of the next larger artery, in its course between the heart and the wound against the nearest bone and thus closing it. Therefore one should press.

1. In bleeding from the forehead the temporal artery just in front of the ear against the temporal bone.

2. In deep bleeding from the neck the carotid artery in the hollow near the larynx against the spinal column. (Fig. 44.)

220   D. Dangers to health from external influences.

3. In bleeding from the shoulder and upper arm the collar bone artery against the first rib; the arms being at the same time firmly drawn down. (Fig. 45.)

4. In bleeding from the arm the artery from the upper arm near the thick flexor muscle against the bone of the upper arm. (Fig. 46.)

5. In bleeding from the upper thigh the artery of the upper thigh in the middle of the groin (§ 7) against the pelvis. (Fig. 47.)

Arterial bleeding from the upper arm and the hand may be stopped by closing the artery of the arm by bending the elbow very forcibly where the pressure

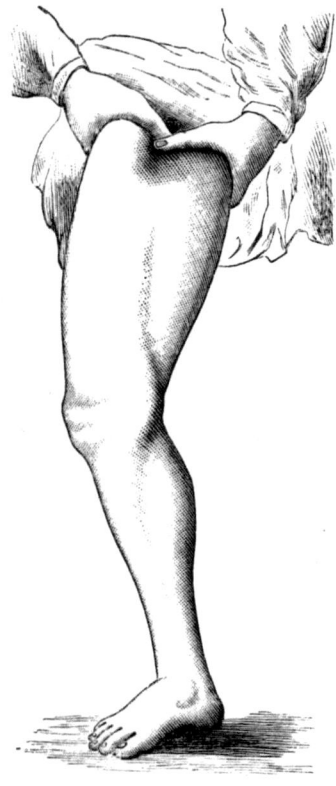

Fig. 47.
Compression of the femoral artery.

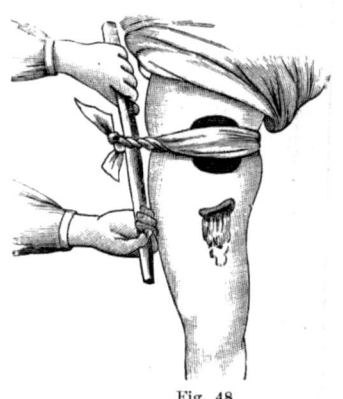

Fig. 48.
A Tourniquet.

of the artery is required for a long time, the easily tired finger is replaced by a hard body (pelotte), e. g. a flat stone, which has been wrapped up in a cloth to prevent contusion of the skin or by a rolled-up bandage. To fasten this pressing body an elastic band is used (braces) or a piece of cloth; this is tied firmly at the side of the limb, opposite to the artery, and is drawn tight by repeatedly twisting a short stick inserted in the knot. (Fig. 48.) A contrivance of this kind is called a *tourniquet* (artery-*press*).

When bleeding from the nose begins, the head should be raised, and the necktie loosened. If the bleeding does not stop soon of its own accord, one should to combat the bleeding by "sniffing" up ice-cold water or vinegar (thinned with water) into the nose or by closing the nostrils with clean wadding. It may also useful to hold up the arms, and to sprinkle the temples repeatedly with cold water. If we do not succed in stopping the bleeding in this manner, medical aid is to be summoned.

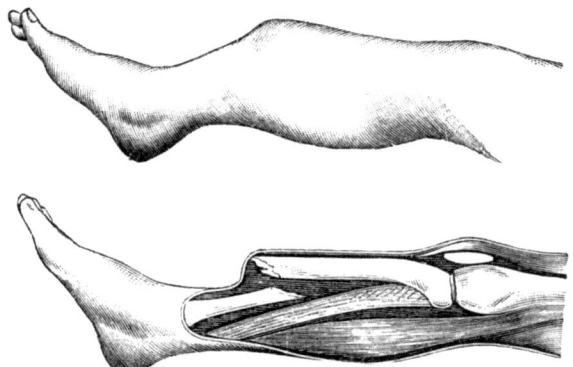

Fig. 49. Broken leg. Etxerior and interior.

Snake bites one should try to suck out; then it is advisable to tie the limb tighthly between the bite and the heart; to cover the wound with cloth, moistened with spirits of wine or of salmiac and to call in a doctor as quickly as possible.

§ 234. **Fractures of bones. Dislocations and sprains.** Bone-fractures are called simple, if the skin over the fracture does not exhibit an open wound; if it does, it is called a compound fracture. As soon as a bone is broke, the part of the body affected, loses its support. One cannot stand on a broken leg, one cannot raise unaided a broken arm; while other injuries may render the movement of the limb difficult on account of pain, but cannot make it altogether impossible. A broken limb appears frequently shortened and thicker in the

D. Dangers to health from external influences.

vicinity of the injury, as the ends of the bone are shifted nearer each other (Fig. 49).

The skin above a fracture usually swells, and assumes a blue colour from extravasated blood. In the effort to lift a broken limb one feels and sometimes hears a crunching of the broken pieces moving against each other, and at the same time we notice an unusual mobility existing in the limb at the point of fracture. The last-mentioned indication of a bone fracture should however be ascertained only by the doctor, entrusted with the treatment of such injuries, as every movement of a broken limb is painful and may injure it.[1]

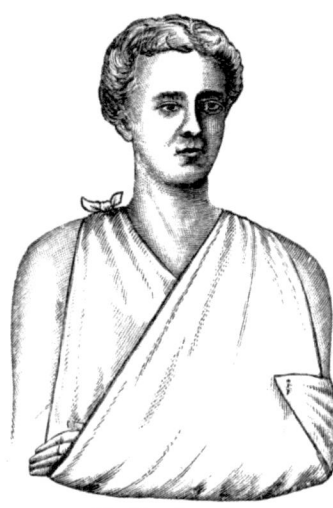

Fig 50. Arm-sling.

Before the arrival of medical aid most benefit is conferred upon the sufferer by insuring rest for the injured member, e. g. by placing a broken leg on a cushion, and supporting it in position by sand-bags, pillows etc.; by fastening a broken upper arm with strings or large cloths to the trunk, and by laying a broken fore-arm in a triangular cloth, slung by two corners round the neck and knotted on the shoulder of the uninjured arm. (Fig. 50). To reduce the swelling and pain it is useful to apply cold-water bandages to the fracture. If it necessary to carry the injured person away (*into his own house or into a hospital*), the broken part should be supported by straight splints, but from wood or strong paste-board, rolled round with some soft material, and fastened with cloths. This protecting apparatus is properly composed of two splints, a longer one fastened on the outside, and a shorter on the inside of the limb. If possible, both splints, and at any rate the outer one should be so long as to project beyond

---

[1] For the purpose of ascertaining the position of broken bones and dislocations surgeons at present make use of the Roentgen rays; also for the purpose of finding strange bodies and for similar purposes.

the two joints nearest to the fracture and to admit of being fastened beyond them. In the case of a fractured leg the sufferer is then placed on a stretcher or in a carriage; care should be taken to protect him from all jolting. In raising patient several persons should lend assistance; one should support exclusively the broken limb by placing one hand above and one hand below the fracture. Any movement of the ends of the broken bones, or any pressure on the seat of the injury should be carefully avoided (cf. also § 256).

In a similar manner as bone fractures dislocations and sprains are treated. *Dislocations* are called all injuries, which cause the starting of a bone from its articulation, mostly by a laceration of the cap of the joint. The power of using the affected joint is withdrawn from the sufferer, or is largely restricted. The neighbourhood of the joint usually becomes more or less swollen; the end of the dislocated bone may be felt in an unusual position and is also visible by the swelling produced; the place, formerly occupied by it appears as a hollow. The setting, i. e. the putting back of the bone into the joint requires skilled knowledge and practice. Any attempt at setting by an unskilled hand causes the sufferer unnecessary pains and may even produce injury.

By *sprains* we understand injuries, arising from a contusion of a joint, or from a tearing of its ligaments, e. g. by inflecting the foot. The joint affected causes pain, when pressed, or when efforts are made to move it; the parts around swell and sometimes it takes long time for them to heal. In sprains, as in other contusions, cold bandages on the injured spot often do good. The same remedy together with a position of complete rest in bed is to be recommended, until the arrival of medical aid in the case of a previously unnoticed *rupture* (cf. § 106) in the abdomen suddenly appears.

§ 235. Burns and corrosions. *Burns* are produced by the action of flames, boiling water, hot objects etc. They are extremely painful and are characterized according to the violence and duration of the heat by redness of the skin, blisters, or complete destruction of the tissues. Burnt parts of the body should be covered by bandages soaked in oil. Burn blisters should not be injured or cut, and in no case should the upper skin prematurely be removed. Only with the employment of dessicating bandages, e. g. of the von Bardeleben (Bismuth) burn-bandage may the blisters be removed with *clean*, previously heated scissors.

Persons, who want to render assistance in fires should wear wet clothes, cover their faces with wet cloths, so that only the eyes remain uncovered. To quench clothes which are burning or smouldering the sufferer should be thrown down upon the ground and covered with blankets, sacks etc. or (in the case of petroleum or spirits of wine) burning with sand, and only afterwards water should be poured upon him.

Similar to burns are *corrosions*, produced by quicklime, acids, alcalies etc. The first help to be given in such cases of injuries should consist in removing the noxious matter from the surface of the body by drying with wadding or cloths. Next the injured part should be washed with water and treated like a burn. Only in cases of quicklime and sulphuric acid water must not be used, as it only increases the corrosive action. Laving with diluted vinegar renders quicklime innocuous; sprinkling with chalk, ashes, soap and magnesia or pouring milk over it renders sulphuric acid innocuous.

About the treatment of persons about to be frozen cf. § 184.

§ 236. Poisoning and intoxication. The symptoms of *poisoning* by the so-called acute poisons are to a very great part those of *corrosion*. By this class of poisons are meant particularly: sulphuric acid (vitriol, oleum) nitric acid (aqua fortis) hydrochloric acid; aqua regia (a mixture of nitric and hydrochloric acid) alcalies and other substances, which, when swallowed cause burning of the mucous membrane of the mouth, alimentary canal and stomach, with which they come in contact. Arsenic is also an acute poison. The nature of the poison taken is often known by the corrosive trace on the lips or in the mouth. Before the arrival of the physician in such cases one may give milk, barley water or gruel and *mild oil* in order to lessen the agony. One should not allow the patient to drink too much water. *Acids* and *alcalies* may be used as remedies against each other, inasmuch as, in *poisoning* from *acids*, innocuous alcaline fluids (such as bicarbonate of soda, or chalk mixed with water) are given to patients; while on the other hand *diluted vinegar* or lemon juice are administered, when *corrosive alcalies* have been swallowed. *Oxalic* *acid poisoning* requires special treatment by lime-water, magnesia or chalk in water.

In case of poisoning by *arsenic* the apothecaries frequently administer a special antidote.

If *phosphorus* has been taken, fatty liquids should not be given to the patient, as these dissolve the poison, and thus facilitate its transfer to the blood. In such cases barley- or water gruel, skimmed milk and a dose of ten drops of ordinary turpentine oil (every half hour to be repeated) should be administered. (The turpentine oil becomes resinous by being exposed to the open air for some time.)

Poisoning by strong, acute vegetable poisons (alcaloids) shows its effect by loss of consciousness and by the contraction of the pupils (morphia and opium) or commencing unrest, excitement, dilatation of the pupils (deadly nightshade, wild cherries) cramps in the muscles increasing to convulsive contractions of the muscles (strychnine). If in such cases of poisoning vomiting has not yet set in, it should be excited, for the purpose of ejecting the poison by trusting the finger deep into the mouth, tickling the throat with the "beard" of a quill-pen or a feather; or by administering any emetic, to be obtained at an apothecary's. The latter however only, if the sufferer has not yet lost consciousness. In cases of opium and morphia poisoning care should be taken, lest the patient falls asleep. Narcotized persons should be brought into a warm room, and be warmed by being wrapped up in woollen blankets. If the face is pale, the head should be placed in a low position; if it is congested, cold bandages round the neck, washing the face and breast or strong emetics are to be employed. If the patient is suffering from difficulty in breathing, artificial respiration should be used (§ 239); but there should in any case be no delay whatever in calling in a doctor, who by anti-dotes, application of the stomach-pump and other remedies frequently averts an unfavourable issue. If the sufferer from poison has not lost consciousness, hot strong coffee or tea should be given to him.

A special kind of poisoning is *intoxication* by over-indulgence in alcoholic drinks, which in extreme cases may also endanger life. It exhibits itself first in fits of excitement of various kinds and gradually leads to complete stupefaction. We should avoid irritating intoxicated persons, and endeavour to remove from them everything, with which they could do injury to themselves or others. If stupefaction has already begun, the intoxication is most easily removed by a long sleep; only, if irregular breathing or other circumstances cause us to suspect danger to life, the treatment recommended for other narcotic poisons should be employed.

§ 237. **Fainting fits and cramps.** By a *fainting fit* we understand the sudden loss of consciousness, which may arise from the effect of bad air, fright, loss of blood, and is sometimes the result of an effusion of blood from the brain. After a preliminary feeling of giddiness and nausea the person affected sinks down suddenly in an insensible condition. One should immediately loosen all clothing round the neck, chest, and abdomen of a person, who has fainted; then he should be laid in an airy place, with his head low, if his face is pale, with his head and upper part of his body raised, if redness of the face indicates congestion of blood in the brain. If the faintness is the result of *a fall or blow on the head*, a position of complete rest, with the upper part of the body raised, should be provided for the injured person.

Good means for reviving persons, who have fainted are: rubbing the forehead with eau de Cologne, and holding strongly smelling substances, such as smelling salts or vinegar, under the nose, using saturated cloths or the moistened hands for that purpose. These liquids should however never be held in a bottle under the nose of the suffering person, as by his movements or by sneezing they might flow into his nose and cause symptoms of choking. In severe fainting fits irritants for the skin, such as rubbing, brushing, and mustard plasters over the heart are very useful. As soon as the fainting person has revived, he should be advised to remain in a lying position quiet for some time still; water or some stimulant should be given to him; a few tea-spoon full of strong wine or coffee or 15 drops of "Hoffmann's drops" in a table-spoon full of water.

Convulsive fits, especially *epileptic convulsions*, which are characterized besides loss of consciousness by contortions of the limbs, rolling of the eyeballs, clenching of the fists etc. must not be confounded with fainting fits. Persons, attacked by convulsions should be placed upon a mattress or quilt; hard or angular objects, against which they might injure themselves, removed from their vicinity and the end of the attack awaited calmly. On the cessation of the convulsions follows frequently sleep of several hours duration, during which the patients are best placed in bed.

§ 238. **Coma.** As *Coma* we designate a state of profound unconsciousness combined with a total cessation of the respiratory movements and utmost lessening of the action of the heart; which state may easily pass into actual death. Its is produced among other causes by drowning, hanging, strangulation, inhalation of poisonous vapours (coal gas, fire damp, carbonic acid in breweries) or of gases, that cannot support life, freezing, heat-stroke, sun-stroke, lightning stroke and action of high tension, electric currents.

In a case of coma, the cause of it must be removed first of all. *Persons, who are taken out of water insensible* should in the first place have all water and mud removed from the mouth and respiratory ways, by laying them on their side and stomach, letting the water run out of their mouth and then cleaning the throat and mouth with the finger, wrapped up in cloth. On no account must such sufferers be placed on their heads for the purpose of letting the water run out. In the case of persons, who have hanged themselves, the rope round the neck should be cut, but care should be taken to support the suspended body, so that it may not receive other injuries by falling down. To sufferers who have *inhaled noxious gases* fresh air should be given directly; the best way is to carry them out into the open air.

§ 239. **Artificial respiration. Conduct in saving from suffocation. Foreign substances in the natural apertures of the body.** The second aid to be given without delay in cases of apparent death is the establishment of *artificial respiration*. The patient should be stripped of all clothes, covering the upper part of the body, and of all garments, confining the body, then laid on his back on the floor on a blanket or mattress and let the back be supported a little by a bundle, which is shoved under it. The tongue is drawn from the mouth and should be held by one of the persons assisting (its slipping back is best prevented by rolling it in a handkerchief) so that in falling back it should not close the larynx. But in case of necessity the tongue is best tied firmly by a string round the lower jaw. The operator then kneels down

228   D. Dangers to health from external influences.

with his knees on either side of the sufferer's hips, and with his hands placed below and to the side of the nipples, the five fingers being laid together and not outstretched, and with his full strength, the ribs against the back and slightly in the direction of the head, so that air audibly escapes from the lungs. This pressure in imitation of expiration is continued for two or three seconds and may be increased by drawing the elbows close to the upper tigh and leaning the upper part of the body forward (Fig. 51).

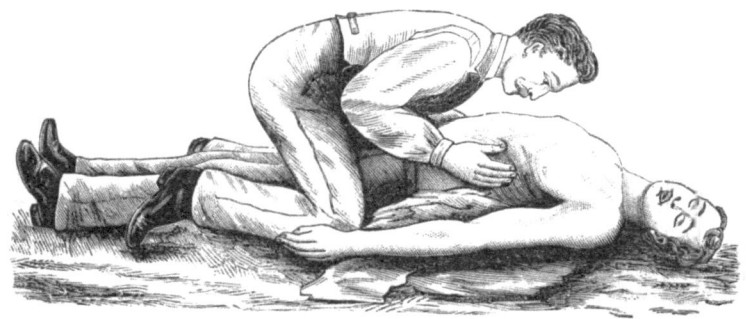

Fig. 51. Artificial respiration. 1. Expiration.

Then the operator suddenly raises himself up, the compressed chest of the sufferer expands on the relaxation of the pressure, and thus causes the lungs to expand also at the same time, by entry of air, as if by natural inspiration (Fig. 52).

After two or three seconds the process commences again; it is repeated ten or twelve times in a minute, and contirued so long, until the natural respiration commences to work again without aid, or until professional, skilled judges opine, that there is no possibility of saving the life of the sufferer, as death has actually taken place.

It is an advantage, if the operator is assisted in his work of saving life by a third person, who kneels at the head of the patient (Fig. 53 and 54) and increases the compression of the chest during expiration by pressing the patient's arms closely against his sides and the expansion of it during inspiration by raising his arms above his head.[1]) As soon as the patient is breathing again, efforts should be made to restore his consciousness by employing the same means, as in cases of fainting.

In cases of giving aid to persons in danger of suffocation, those engaged in the work of rescue should observe certain precautions for their own safety. Before entering

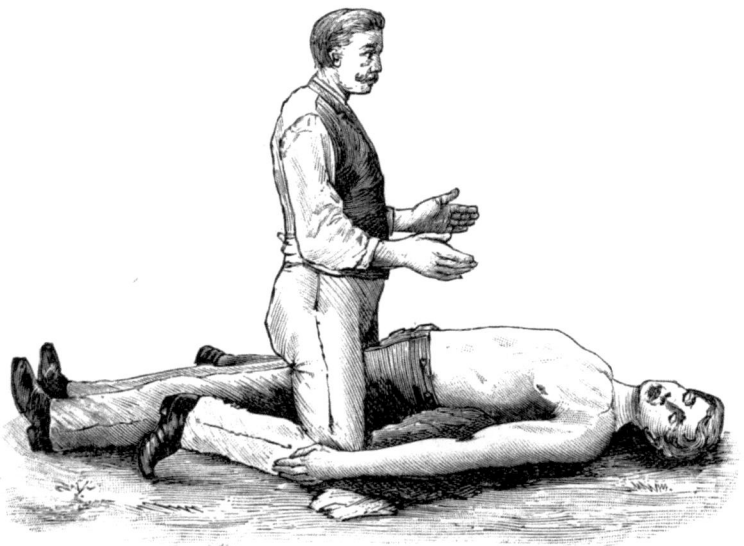

Fig. 52. Artificial respiration. I. Inspiration.

rooms, filled with noxious gases care should be taken to air them completely by opening the doors wide, and breaking in the windows from the outside. If the latter is impossible, the rescuer should hold a cloth, moistened with water or diluted vinegar before his mouth, hasten through the room and go to the sufferer only, after the air has been cleared out and a complete draught of air established. If suffocating persons are to lifted out of wells, shafts, pits, sewers, canals, deep

---

[1]) This procedure cannot be employed, if the bones or the chest of the sufferer have been injured or broken, as for instance in cases of caving in of earth etc.

230   D. Dangers to health from external influences.

cellars etc., the rescuer in descending should have a rope fastened round his body, so that in case of emergency he might be taken out at once, moreover communiction should be

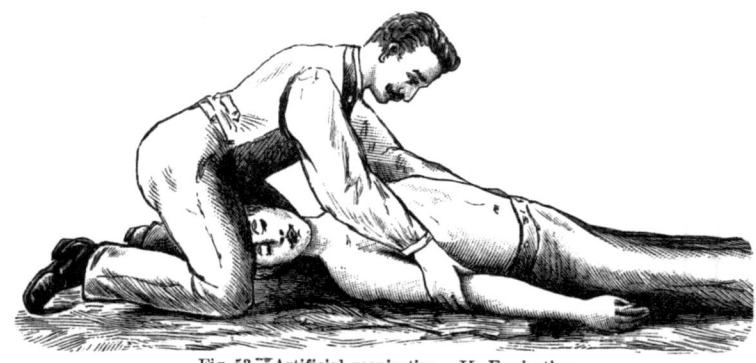

Fig. 53. Artificial respiration. II. Expiration

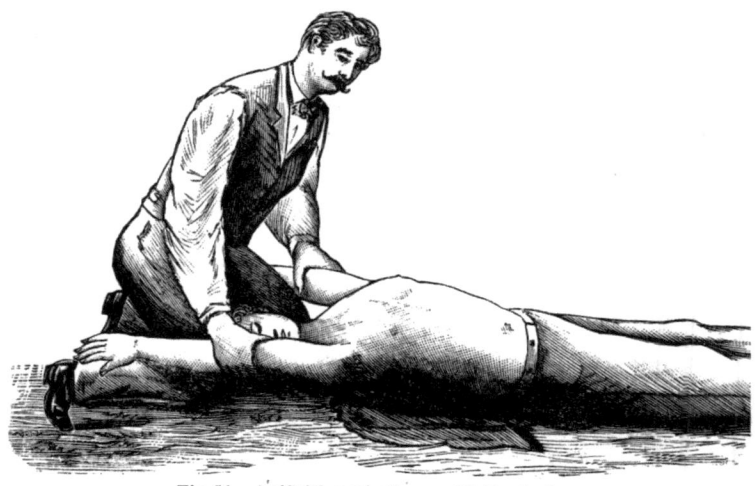

Fig. 54. Artificial respiration. II. Inspiration.

maintained with the outer world by means of a line, fastened to the arm, by pulling of which a signal may be given, in case danger requires the rescuer to be drawn up. If the noxious gas in such cases consists of carbonic acid, it may be made more or less harmless by pouring whitewash down. One should never enter rooms, suspected of containing escaped gas with a light; in such gases the main cock and all other open gas-cocks should be turned off at once.

In rescuing persons, *buried* under falls of *rubbish* etc. care should be taken not to suffer from caving in of masses of earth etc. The injured should be lifted up carefully, because his bones might be broken. To facilitate his breathing the earth, which has got into his mouth should be removed with a wrapped up finger.

Danger of suffocation sometimes occurs as the result of *swallowing of foreign, substances,* such as bones, fish bones etc. One should try to remove such objects with the wrapped up finger; but to avoid the risk of being bitten in doing so, a broad piece of wood should be placed between the teeth of the sufferer. If the foreign substance cannot be removed in this way, the result may be obtained by pressure upon the belly, strong blows on the back, or an incitement to vomiting (§ 236). If the substance is not sticking in the windpipe, but in the gullet, it may be forced down with a bread crumb or a fatty morsel and thus pass into the stomach. In serious cases, by which life is endangered the surgeon may procure help by the employment of special instruments, and in extreme danger by tracheotomy (incision in the windpipe).

Medical aid must be called, if *foreign objects*, insects etc. find ingress into the ear, eye, nose or *other apertures of the human body*, an accident sometimes occurring with children.

If the effort to remove these objects is not successful at once, the non professional person should stop his efforts, because serious injury may be done by too violent pulling, tearing or piercing.

For the treatment of sun stroke, heat stroke and lightning see § 185. Persons who are injured by *artificial electric currents* should be treated like persons struck by lightning.

Supplement.

Preliminary knowledge for nursing the sick.

§ 240. Importance of nursing. By following the rules of hygiene, we may restrict the number of illnesses and accidents, but we cannot completely prevent them. There will be always sick and injured persons, who desire to have their health restored, or their pains alleviated, and who require the care of their fellow-men.

In general, the healing of the sick and wounded is the business of the *medical man*. For the correct diagnosis of a malady, the decision about the proper way of healing and nursing; the laying down of rules, to be observed by the patients must be based upon exact knowledge of the parts and functions of the body, as well as familiarity with the morbid deviations from the usual and an accurate knowledge of the modus and the effect of all known healing methods. The knowledge, necessary for this purpose cannot be acquired without years of laborious study under professional tuition; the correct application is insured only by accumulated experience.

Besides the advice and aid of the physician however *careful nursing* is of great importance in the course and for the result of the illness, as well as for alleviating the pains, connected with it. It is not always possible to entrust the patients to trained male or female nurses; anyone may be placed in a position of having to undertake the duty of nursing in person, should anyone under our care fall ill. No one should therefore delay to make himself acquainted with the essential duties to be done in such cases.

If limited means and domestic relations make nursing difficult in one's own house, it is advisable to remove the patient to a hospital. The more perfect the arrangements of such institutions, which have constantly on hand trained nurses and doctors ready to give assistance afford the best possible guarantee for recovery (§ 145).

§ 241. **The sick-room.** The first necessity in nursing the sick is the preparing of a *suitable sick-room*. The patient requires quiet before all things; a room as isolated as possible, and one, which is not at the same time occupied by healthy persons should be provided; and should the doctor consider it necessary, no one should enter it, except the persons entrusted with the treatment and nursing of the patient. The room should be large enough, so as to afford space for plenty of fresh air; daylight should have abundant access to it, and there should be good means for lighting up the room in the evening and during the night. However; there should be some means of darkening the room and of protecting the patient by screens, curtains etc. from too glaring light and from the heat of the sun. If a room is used as a sick room in winter, care should be taken that it has a good heating apparatus, capable of maintaining a temperature of 15^0 to 17^0 C.

Special attention should be paid to *cleanliness* in the sick-room (§ 229 f. 3). Objects, likely to retain dust and unnecessary furniture, which both make the room small and increase the difficulty of cleaning it should be removed. The floor should be swept every day with as little discomfort to the patient as possible, and should be scrubbed now and then. The room should be aired every morning and evening and each time the patient had an evacuation of the bowels. The remains of food, utensils, which have been used, excretions, dirty under-linen and bed-clothing etc. should not be tolerated in the sick-room, but should be immediately removed, if necessary after previous disinfection or after other means of precaution have been employed for the prevention of propagation of any infection germs.

§ 242. **The sick-bed.** The *sick-bed* is best placed in such a position, that it touches only with one end (where the head of the patient is) the wall; all the others sides should be freely accessible. It should be neither exposed to the direct heat from the stove, nor to a troublesome draught from the door or window, and, if necessary, should be protected by large bed-screens. It should be of sufficient size, and be provided with good bedding; mattresses, stuffed with horse-hair should be used to lie upon. The bed-linen should be always clean, and must be therefore frequently changed. In cases, where the patients soil the bed-linen with their evacuations, the mattress should be protected by an india-rubber sheet. To support the head, or, if necessary, the upper part of the body well-stuffed cushions, which however should not be too soft should be used. As covering woollen blankets are recommended; in some cases light feather-beds may be used, if the patient has been used to them; but in no case should too heavy or too many coverings be employed.

As a rule, the patient finds himself most comfortable, when he lies *on his back*, with his *head* somewhat *raised*. In cases of difficulty of breathing, the upper half of the body should be raised by pillows, or by a stool, placed with its back against the pillow. To prevent the patient from gliding down, his feet should be placed against a hard cushion or a block of wood. Patients, who are too weak to raise themselves alone, find a cord attached to the foot of the bed useful, with a wooden cross-handle as lever, to raise themselves in bed. Against the feeling of frost the best remedy are heated stones or *warming pans*, i. e. either well-closed metal pans or stone jars, filled with hot water. These vessels are placed in the bed next to the patient; but they should be wrapped in cloths, so as not to touch the skin of the patient. The bed should frequently be smoothed down under the patient; and also cleared of bread-crumbs, sand and similar things. If the patient cannot leave the bed for the time necessary to do his bed up, he should be removed to another bed or sopha (§ 256). The bed should be warmed, if necessary, before the patient is brought back to his newly-made bed.

§ 243. Care of the patient's body. Bedsores. Great attention should be paid to the patient *cleanliness* and *nursing of his body*. Weakly patients should be washed on hands and face and if necessary on other parts of the body with warm water at least twice a day by the nurse, who should use a soft sponge. The hair should be combed at the same time.

The patient should also daily clean his teeth and rinse his mouth; in cases of patients, who cannot do this themselves, the nurse should rub their mouths from time to time with a damp cloth. To feverish persons it is often refreshing to have their dry lips rubbed with mild oil or ointment.

A frequent change of linen is advantageous for all sick people, especially for those, who perspire. The change of linen should be effected only, when perspiration has ceased, and the patient's skin has been dried under the bed-clothes with warm cloths. A change of shirt is best carried out by opening all buttons under the bed-cloths, slipping the shirt from under the patient by gently raising him, and then quickly, but carefully pulling it over his head and arms. The fresh shirt, *which should be previously warmed*, is then slipped in the same way over the head and arms, and drawn down as smooth as possible under the bed clothes.

By attention to cleanlines and conscientious management not only is the comfort of the patient promoted, but they are also the necessary conditions for preventing the dreaded *bed-sore*. In the case of weak patients confined to bed for a long time, the parts of the body, on which they principally lie, the heels, loins, os sacrum and the region of the shoulder-blades easily become sore. First appear redness and sensitiveness of the skin; then sore spots are observed, which quickly increase in size and become deeper, causing the patient much uneasiness and may become dangerous, by causing blood-poisoning. Such undesirable results are inevitable in the case of some diseases, if the body, as well as the under and bed-linen of the patient is not kept scrupulously clean, and if diligent attention is not paid, to keep the ticking smooth and free from creases. As soon as a bed-sore has developed, its healing occasions great difficulties, as the patient is compelled to lie further on the same spot. Therefore the sick nurse should take particular conscientious care to notice red or painful spots upon the recumbent portions of the body, and to call in a doctor, as soon as they show themselves. Frequently it is advantageous to moisten the skin, when red with lemon-juice, camphorated wine or French brandy; but it is especially advisable in tedious long-lasting cases of illness to lay *air-beds* or *water-beds* on the mattress, as bed-sores are not so easily developed on such supports.

§ 244. Watching by the sick. Conduct of the nurse. A nurse should be constantly present with patients seriously ill, in order to observe them, and to hand them anything, which they may require. Expecially excited and delirious persons require constant watching, so as to be restrained from actions, which may cause injury to themselves and others. In such cases the nurse should restrain the patient with calm and moderate words from senseless actions; but otherwise and in everything follow strictly the directions of the doctor; he should report to the latter at his next visit all his observations in regard to the conduct of the patient. If the doctor has ordered night watching, a change of the nursing staff for the day and for the night should be provided, so the nurse should have time to rest sufficiently, before beginning his duties.

The nurse should do his duties quietly and noiselessly; should not worry the patient with his own uncertainty, anxiety or troubles, and should be as gentle as possible in giving assistance. In the care of such persons, who suffer from infectious diseases, the nurse should avoid eating or drinking or putting his fingers to his mouth while in the sick-room. After touching the patient, the hands should be washed with soap and a brush: when leaving the sick-room the clothing should be changed, if possible. It is advisable, while remaining with the patient, to wear an apron or similar garment of washing material over the whole clothing.

§ 245. Sleep and breathing of the patient. As a rule the nurse should not disturb the patient's *sleep*. In cases, where too long a sleep would be injurious, or where the patient must be awakened, e. g. to take medicine or at mealtime, the doctor will give orders to that effect. A well-aired toom, a freshly made bed, soft light and for feverish patients cooling drinks facilitate the patient's falling asleep.

The nurse should pay attention to the patient's *breathing*, to be able to report later on, whether it was rapid or slow, difficult or painful, accompanied by groans and movement of the nostrils. Should rattling in the chest cause the nurse to suspect an accumulation of phlegm in the air-passages, the patient should be put up sitting from time to time, to facilitate his coughing it up. The patient should be advised, *not to swallow his expectorations*, but to spit into a spitting vessel, which the nurse holds with the one hand, while the other holds the pillow under his head and supports the upper part of the body in a sitting position. The expectoration should be kept until the next visit of the doctor, in order to be shown to him and rendered innocuous or removed according to his directions.

§ 246. **Bleeding.** Special help is necessary in case of much bleeding from the mouth. This comes generally from the lungs, if it is accompanied by coughing, and if the blood is of bright-red colour, mixed with air-bubbles. Vomited blood on the other hand is usually of a dark-red colour, and arises from a blood-vessel in the stomach having been opened by an ulcerating process. In every case of violent bleeding it is necessary to call the doctor immediately; but until his arrival the patient should be kept as quietly as possible on his back, with the upper part of his body raised; all talking should be forbidden to him, and according to the supposed locality of the bleeding the chest or stomach should be kept cool by ice-cold bandages or by an ice-bladder (§ 253). On the occurrence of internal bleeding, which can be recognized by the sudden corpse-like pallor of the patient, the same precautions should be taken for a quiet position of the patient and for the immediate summoning of the doctor.

§ 247. **Heart-beat; Pulse; Temperature of the body.** It is frequently useful to observe the *heart-beat* of the patient; to count his *pulse* from time to time, and to take the *temperature* of his body, so as to be able to report to the doctor regularly the result of such observations from notes, made at the time. The temperature of the body is best measured by the so-called *clinical thermometer*, divided into tenths of degrees. (The best is the so-called maximal-thermometer.) This is placed with the mercury bulb in the carefully dried hollow under the arm of the invalid; the latter is requested to hold his arm close to his body, for which in cases of weakness or delirium the assistance of the nurse is necessary and after ten minutes the height of the thermometer is ascertained by observation of the mercury column. After two minutes more, note is taken, whether the mercury has risen still further. If this is not the case, the measuring can be interrupted; otherwise, it has to be continued so long, until within two minutes more no further rise takes place. Before every reading one should ascertain, whether the mercury stands already above

36° C. By swinging the thermometer up and down, a sinking of the mercury may be effected.

§ 248. Natural excretions of the patient. Injections and enemas. At the order of the doctor, or as soon as the *urine* and *excreta* of the patient exhibit unusual characteristics, these excreta must be preserved (outside the sickroom), if they do not take place at the regular time, this fact also must be notified to the doctor. Patients, who cannot or dare not leave the bed, should have the pan (warmed) placed under them, and the urine-glass placed before them. During evacuation the patient is to be supported by the nurse. If the linen is soiled accidentally, it should be replaced immediately by clean linen. In order to avoid as far as possible such occurrences with patients, who pass their excreta involuntarily, the vessels, intended for their reception should be placed under them, unasked from time to time. Patients, who get up for the closet or to urine should be protected against catching cold by being well wrapped up by warm clothing.

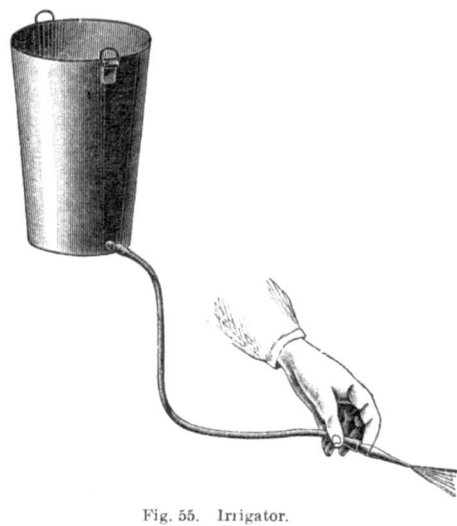

Fig. 55. Irrigator.

To *stimulate* the action of the bowels *injections* by means of *syringes* sold for that purpose, or, better enemas by means of the so-called irrigator are administered, the fluid being thus either forced in, or allowed to flow into the rectum. In purchasing instruments for this purpose, care should be taken, that the nozzle of the syringe or irrigator is rounded and made of flexible material (hard india-rubber) so that no injury may be caused to the rectum by its insertion. These instruments should never be used without being previously thoroughly cleaned. The operation itself is performed in the following manner. The patient is laid on his side; a vessel being placed alongside him on the bed previously protected against wetting by a waterproof sheet, and is supported in this position by placing a hand on the back; with the other hand the nozzle of the syringe or irrigator is carefully inserted in the orifice, and then by gentle, constant pressure on the piston of the syringe or by moderate lifting of the irrigator the liquid is allowed to run in. Unless the doctor orders otherwise, the liquid, used for on injection should consist of about $\frac{3}{4}$ litre of tepid water with an addition of one or two teaspoon full of salt. The effect of the injection or enema is all the more certain, the longer the liquid is retained by the patient.

§ 249. Vomiting. Attention to bandages. Nourishment of the invalid. When vomiting the patient is to be assisted by raising and supporting his head (§ 245). He should be induced to suppress the inclination to vomit, because the actual vomiting is thereby shortened and the unpleasant retching is in some degree lessened. When the vomiting is over, the mouth and nose should be cleaned. It is also well to refresh the patient with cooling drinks in small quantities. The vomit itself must be kept until the arrival of the doctor.

The nurse must keep a particularly watchful eye on the temporary bandages of the patient. Any disturbances, which appear must be skilfully removed. If a sudden redness or saturation of the bandage with blood announces an increased bleeding the surgeon should be informed at once. Until his arrival the directions of § 233 are to be observed.

Of great importance for the well-being of the patient is the modus of his *nourishment*. Disobedience of the doctor's orders may occasionally exercise a highly prejudicial influence on the course of the disease (cf. § 202). In public hospitals strict measures are taken, that visitors from without should not bring improper food and dainties to the patients. As a rule, at the beginning of an illness it is well to give only slops (liquid food) to the patient, before the doctor arrives; these slops include milk; thin barley or oaten gruel with an addition of some meat broth, but the patient should not be forced to partake of this food. Cooled boiled water with some lemon-juice and sugar can be recommended as a refreshing beverage.

§ 250. Giving of medicine. All *remedies* must be *admini-*

stered strictly according to the prescription at definite times and in measured quantities. *Liquid remedies* are best kept cool by placing them in a vessel, partly filled with water. At each dose the medicine, after shaking the bottle should be poured into a spoon or wineglass, previously well cleaned and brought to the patient's mouth, who is at the same time supported in a sitting position. *Pills* or *capsules* are most easily swallowed down with a mouthful of water. *Powders* are best mixed in a spoon with some water, unless it is preferred to administer in *wafers*. A wafer about 6 cm in diameter is moistened on a plate, and the powder shaken on it; it is then rolled in the form of a ball, and swallowed by the patient with some water on it. The use of force in administering medicines to refractory patients is permissible only in rare cases, to be determined by the doctor (for instance with children).

Unfortunately a *mistake* in giving the *wrong bottle* has frequently led to accidents; we should therefore always satisfy ourselves before giving it by reading the inscription on the label attached to the medicine bottle, so as to exclude the possibility of mistakes. The self-administration of medicines should never be permitted to seriously sick persons.

§ 251. **Painting. Massage. Embrocation.** *Painting, embrocations* and *massage* are to be carried out strictly according to the doctor's orders. *Massage*, like a number of other operations, necessary in nursing the sick, e. g. leeching, cupping etc. requires some practice, and should therefore be left to trained persons. Skilfully executed, it may prove very beneficial in many cases; e. g. in removing swellings in the joints, or in restoring flexibility in the limbs after the union of fractured bones. As its application in unsuitable cases may also have injurious effects, this treatment should only be applied in pursuance on the doctor's orders.

Anybody may be safely entrusted with the *application* of *embrocations*. The liquids or ointments, ordered for this purpose are rubbed on the surface of the body either with the fingertips, or the ball of the thumb, or the whole palm of the hand, with a circular motion and a pressure, sometimes gentle, sometimes strong, but always uniform.

§ 252. **Mustard-plasters and blisters.** Sometimes *mustard-plasters or blisters* are ordered for the patient. Instead of the former, the mustard paper (to be bought) is recently much used. This is moistened on the coated side, and laid for ten or fifteen minutes on the portion of the skin, marked by the doctor; after its removal, the skin, which will be very red, if the plaster has acted, must be washed with a soft sponge and warm water. *Spanish-fly paper* is used for blisters. It is similarly moistened, and kept on from twelve to twenty four hours, in each case, until a blister has formed on the place. After its removal, the blister is "pricked" open with a needle (which has been heated red-hot, and cooled again) and is dressed with ointment as soon as the liquid has flowed out. Any dirt is to be carefully avoided, as the part of the skin under the blister is to be considered as a wound.

In applying mustard-plasters and blisters those portions of the skin, on which the patient lies, e. g. joints and particularly sensitive parts of the body, as the nipples and navel must not be selected. Great care must be taken with spanish-fly blisters, as the ingredient, to which their effect is due, is very poisonous.

§ 253. Ice-bags. Cold bandages. As *ice-bags* bladders are used, made of impenetrable substances, — the best are from india-rubber, — and capable of being well closed. These are filled with ice, broken to pieces, the size of a hazelnut or walnut, by wrapping a large piece in a cloth and smashing it with a hammer. The ice-bag is laid as broad as possible on the spot, indicated by the doctor. It should be wrapped in a linen cloth, because the watertight material easily lets through some humidity, and then its dampness is very uncomfortable for the patient. In many cases, as when laying the ice-bag on the head, it may be fastened by a string too the bedpost, so that it can neither ship off, nor press to heavily.

Where an ice-bag cannot be had, an effort is made to replace it by *cold bandages*. A handkerchief or napkin, folded several times is laid on a piece of ice or in the coldest possible water wrung out well after some time, and applied to the part of the body, to be cooled. As a bandage of this kind heats quickly on the skin, it must be frequently changed; in some cases, every minute.

§ 254. Cold douches and swathings. Moist-warm bandages. Dry heat. While ice-bags and cold bandages have in view a longer or shorter cooling, the effect of *cold douches and* *swathings* partly rests on the fact, that the blood driven out of the skin by the cold afterwards flows back again in increased quantity. In this way circulation as well as the excretory functions of the skin and kidneys is stimulated, and a pleasant heat produced in the body. Unless this method is employed in healthy persons in order to "harden" themselves it should never be used without medical advice, as such cures may be injurious in the cases of some patients

A lasting increase of the blood, contained in the skin is effected by *moist warm or hydropathic (Prießnitz) bandages*. They consist in wrapping or covering the skin with wet muslin *(not dripping with water)* or moist linen, which is prevented from drying up by an envelope of water-proof material, and is fastened by strings or cloths. Whether cold or warm water is used for damping the bandage is immaterial, as the heat of the body soon communicates itself to it.

In some cases use is also made of dry heat in the treatment of patients by fastening to the surface of the body heated cloth or heated sacks, filled with sand, bran, chaff or herbs. Such appliances are popular among other things against *toothache*. But for this purpose frequent rinsing of the mouth with hot camomile tea is more effective.

§ 255. Baths. Sweating cures. Baths are extensively used in sick-nursing. We distinguish between full baths and local baths; such as half baths, hip baths, arm baths, hand baths and foot baths. The bath water is used sometimes hot 36 to 40^0 C.), sometimes warm ($31—35^0$ C.), lukewarm ($26—30^0$ C.), cool ($21—25^0$ C.) or cold ($16—20^0$ C.). According to the order of the physician either ordinary water is used, or water from curative springs. The addition of salt or other ingrediences is often useful. The opinion of a doctor should first be obtained as to the kind and duration of every bath, as well as the douches etc. frequently taken in connection with the bath. Sometimes *hot-air* baths (Roman) or *steam baths* (Russian) are ordered; but such baths as a rule should be taken only in special bathing establishments. If baths are to be taken by patients seriously ill, it is advisable to have strong wine at hand, as weakness sometimes occurs in the bath. Immediately after the bath the patient should be quickly dried and dressed, or be put back in bed. Bathing vessels, used by infectious patients should be disinfected. In case it is intended, that the patient should perspire after the bath, he is completely wrapped and well covered in with a woollen sheet. When the perspiration is over, he should be treated in the manner indicated in § 243.

Sometimes it is sought to stimulate perspiration by hot drinks. The kinds of tea, used for this purpose, (elder tea, linden blossom tea) are prepared by putting a certain quantity of the substance into a well-warmed vessel filled with boiling water, and then straining it through a sieve or clean linen cloth.

§ 256. Transport of the sick. If it is necessary to transport the patient to other rooms, he must be protected by suitable wrappings against catching cold. In lifting and carrying him, two persons must lend assistance; of whom one supports the legs, while the other grasps the patient under the cross and by the shoulder, the patient clasping the latter round the neck. For the removal of patients from one house to another, either stretchers or carriages with good springs should be used. In case of necessity a door taken off its hinges, a large sack, supported by poles on either side, or a ladder covered with a mattress, can be used as stretchers. Carriages should drive carefully, if necessary at a walking pace.

Index.

(The number refers to the page.)

Abdomen 7.
— Pancreas 21.
— Peritoneum 21.
— Peritonitis 200. 201.
Abdominal cavity 10.
— inflammation 201.
— Typhoid 191. 192.
Abscess 205.
Accidents 217.
— on railways and ships 145.
— insurance 167.
— insurance of workmen 166. 167.
— annuity 168.
— in factories 167. 168.
Acclimatization 175.
Acetylene gas 124.
Acids (of the vegetable kingdom) 90.
— poisoning by 224.
Actinomyces 84.
Actinomycosis 84.
Action of cells 22. 23.
Action of the bowels 238.
Activity
— of the brain 128.
Air 35.
— dryness 119.
— heat of 37. 38.
— movement 39. 40.
— necessity of fresh for children 151.
— moisture of 37. 38.
— beds 235.
— contamination 41.

Air impurities 137.
— pressure 40. 41.
— space for — in dwellings 114.
— windpipe 13.
Albumin 55. 56.
— ous bodies 56.
— foods 21.
Alcalies
— poisoning by 224.
Alcaloids (vegetable kingdom poisons) 225.
Alcohol 93.
— Indulgence in and disadvantage of 93. 96. 97. 129.
— poisoning by 225.
Aluminium vessels 101.
Anæmia 214.
Anchylostomum duodenale 214.
Aneroïd barometer 40.
Animal's diseases 207.
— contagious 207.
— carcases 144.
— removal of 144.
Anthrax
— bacillus 208.
— carbuncle 208.
— modes of propagation 166.
Antidote 225.
Aorta 16.
Apothecaries 141.
Apples (American) 74.
Arak 96.

Arc-electric light 124.
Argand-burner 114. 123.
Argon 35.
Armpit 11.
Arm-sling 222.
Arms, broken arms, see bones broken 7. 11.
Army
— illness in 2.
— infectious diseases in 179.
Arsenic, poisoning by 166.
Arteries 15. 16.
Artesian well 46.
Artichokes 70.
Artificial eating fat 89.
— law concerning it 89. 140.
— wine 94.
Asparagus 70.
Assemblies
— of human beings 140.
Astralagus 12.
— Tarsus 12.
Atmosphere 35.
Auricle (right and left) 15.

Bacilli 176.
Back 7.
— spinal marrow 25 to 28.
— spinal nerves 27.
Backbone 10.
— spinal curvature 156.
Bacon 89.

Index.

Bacteria 176. 177.
Bake-ware 64.
Baking powder 65.
Ball of the little finger 11.
Bananas 73.
Bandages 239.
— aseptic (antiseptic) 204.
— cold 241. 242.
Barbel cholera 90.
Barley 67. 95.
— Pearl 67.
— sugar 74.
Barometer 40.
Baths 53. 151. 242.
— Hot-air (Roman) 242.
— steam (Russian) 242.
— shower 54.
Beans 68. 70.
Bed 108.
— pan 238.
Bedroom 114.
Bedsore 234. 235.
Beer 95.
Beet-sugar 56. 74.
Belly 7.
Belt 106.
Berries 73.
Beverages
— alcoholic 93.
— injurious to school-children 158.
Bismuth
— dessicating 223.
— bandages 223.
Bitters 96.
Black bread 65.
Black death 179. 202.
Bleeding
— Arterial 220.
— Remedies for stopping 218. 237.
Blisters 108.
Blood 4. 15.
— Change in colour of 15.
— Venes and arteries 15. 16.
— Corpuscles of 15.
— Circulation of 15—18.
— Disturbances in circulation of 18. 107.

Blood vessels 4. 15.
— spitting 210.
— coughing 210.
— disorders in the formation of 213. 214.
Body 4—6.
— Aorta 16.
— circulation (of the blood) 17.
— cleaning 52. 53.
— development in school 159.
— heat of 23, 237.
— neglect of 149.
— position in different trades 164.
Boil, purulent 205.
Bone-
— Heel 12.
— hyoid 9.
Bones 4.
— fractures 221.
Boots, shoes 107.
Bovine tuberculosis 77. 212.
Brain 6. 25—27.
— Great 26.
— little 26.
— Apoplexy 27.
— Inflammation of cerebral membrane 201. 213.
— nerves 27.
Bran
— bread 65.
Brandy 96. 97.
— Injury to health 97.
— Different kinds of 96.
Brass utensils 100.
Breathing 12—14.
Bread 64—66.
— Baking of 64.
— basket 101.
— Green-bread-basket 101.
Breast 7.
Brightness 122.
Brown bread (rye-bread) 65. 66.
Buck-wheat 68.
Building materials 109.
— for roofs 112.

Building ground 109.
— subsoil 110.
Building police regulation
— of Berlin 112. 127. 137.
Bulbons, vegetables 101.
Burial places 142.
Burns 235.
Butter 56. 79.
— Surrogates of 79. 80. 140.
— Laws referring to 140.
— Preserved 79.

Cabbage 70.
Caecum 20.
— Inflammation of 20.
Cakes, Confectionery 75.
— Sweet stuffs 75.
Calf of the leg 12.
— fibula 12.
Cancer 215. 216.
Candles 122.
Cane sugar 56. 74.
Cannon-stove 117.
Capillary vessels 16.
— Care of the hair 53.
Carbo-hydrates 55.
Carbolic soap (Cresol) 181.
— solution 218.
Carbonic acid.
— of the air 35. 36.
— in the blood 19.
— natron stove 118.
— poisonous nature of 36. 37.
Carbuncle 204. 205.
Caries 210.
Carpets 113.
Carrots 70.
Cartage 132.
— of human excreta 125.
Cartilage 4.
Casein 55. 76. 80.
— Law concerning 140.
Cataract 30.
Catarrh 171.
Caviare 91.
Cellar
— dwelling in 110. 113. 127.

Cellulose 56.
Central heating 116.
Cerebral membranes
— tuberculosis of 210.
Cess-pools 125. 132.
Champagne wine 94.
Cheek bones 7.
Cheeks 7.
Cheese
— Kinds of 80.
Chervil 70.
Chewing tobacco 99.
Chicken-pox 185. 190.
Chill blains 172.
Chimney 117.
— top (ventilating) 115.
— (mantle piece) 116.
Chin 7.
Chlorosis 214.
Chocolate 98.
Choice of profession 161.
— precautionary measures against accidents 166. 167.
Cholera 194—196.
— Asiatic 194.
— Prevention of the Propagation of 148. 195.
— Modus of living during 196.
— Typhoid 195.
— nostras 194.
Choroid 28.
Chyme 22.
Circulation-stove 119.
Cistern 44.
Clarifying vessels 49.
Cleanliness clothing and bedding 110.
Clearing process 134.
Climate
— change of 42. 174.
Closets
— disinfection 126.
Closure of frontiers 147.
— of shops 163.
Clothes 23. 102—105.
— fastening of 105.
— form of 105—107.
— too tight 105—107.
Clouds 39.

Coal
— gas 116. 118. 123. 124.
Cocci 176.
Cocoa 97.
— butter 69. 98.
Coffee 97.
— adulteration of 98.
— artificial 140.
— disadvantage of drinking 99.
— substitutes 98.
Cognac, see Brandy 96.
Cold swathings 241, 242.
— moist-warm 242.
— Priessnitz 242.
— influence of 170.
— s through wetting 103.
— protection against 171.
Collar bone 10. 11.
Collecting basin 45.
Collective heating 116.
— by steam 120.
— advantage of 120. 121.
Colonial molasses 74.
Colours
— change in colour of 16.
— injurious to heath 140.
Coma 172. 237.
Comma-bacilli 176.
Commerce and means of communication 144.
Compensation for damages 168.
Concert halls 141.
Condiments (spices) 58. 92.
Conjunctiva 31.
Constituents soluble, of the soil 44.
Consciousness
— Seat of 27.
Contusion 223.
— wounds 218.
Convulsions 227.
Cooking 58.
— salt 91. 92.
— utensils 100. 101.

Cooking vessels 100. 101.
Copper vessels 100.
Corium 6.
Corn 63.
— Kind of 66. 67.
Cornea 28. 29.
— spots of 206.
Corns 108.
Corpse
— burial 142.
— of persons, who died of infectious diseases 143. 144.
— Inspection of 143.
Corrosions 223.
Corset 106. 107.
Cotton stuffs 103. 104.
— seed oil 69. 80.
Cranberries 73.
Cray fish
— poisoning by 91.
Cream, formation of 77. 78.
Crisis 184.
Cristalline lens 28.
Crooked position of children 156. 157.
Croup, Diphtherie 197.
Crown on the top cf the head 6.
Crustacea 91.
— poisoning by 91.
Cucumbers 70.
Curly cabbage 70.
— taverns frequenting of 129.
Cysts 84.

Deadly nightshade 225.
Deep pump well 45.
Delirium tremens 97.
Deposits
— atmospheric (rain, snow, hail) 39.
— water 43. 44.
Disinfection 141. 180. 183.
— of goods 148.
— of clothes and luggage of travellers 147.
— houses 182.
— means of 181. 182.

Destruction of germs 180. 181.
— in case of infectious disease 180. 181.
Diabetes 214.
Diaphragm 10.
Diarrhœa 171. 193.
Diastase 95.
Diet
— Calculation of daily 58. 61—63.
— change of 58.
— vegetarian 56.
Digestible
— food 63.
Digestion 21—23.
— Organs of 19.
Dill 92.
Diphtheria 197—199.
— healing serum 198.
Dirt, removal by water 51. 52.
Disease
— Course of 183.
— germs 41. 176.
— infection 101. 146. 147.
— interstices of dwellings 113.
— prevention of propagation 101. 146. 147.
— preventive measures in schools 159.
— propagation of 101. 146. 147.
— vitality of in corpses 142. 143.
— Foot and mouth 77. 208.
— Bright's 153.
Dislocation 223.
Dispersion of smoke (for smoking tobacco) 137.
Distilling 51.
Douches 54. 242.
— cold 241.
Drainage 132.
— and drying of the house 111. 112.
Draught 115. 171.
— on railways 146.
Draw-wells 46.

Drinking vessels 100.
— water 43.
Drugbook of German Empire 141.
Duodenum (twelve finger intestine) 20.
Duration of daily work 162.
Dust 41. 42. 135.
— diseases 165.
Dwellings 109.
— Utilization of 114.
— hight 114.
— space 114.
— keeping cool of 122.
— cleanliness of 125.
— plan of 114.
— articles for use in 127.
Dysentery 196 197.
— of the infantile period 151.

Ear 7. 32. 33.
— External 32.
— middle 32.
— inner 32.
— shell 32.
— wax 32.
— Tympanun 32.
— cocklea 32.
— Eustachian canal 32.
Earthenware stoves 119 to 121.
Echinococcus (Dog-Tapeworm) 216.
Edible cockless
— mussels 91.
Education 149.
Eggs 81.
— conservation of 81.
— of a hen 81.
Elbow-joint 11. 27.
Electric current
— accidents by means of 231.
Embrocations 240.
Emetic 225.
Endemic 178.
Endive salad 70.
Enema 238.
Epidemics 178.

Epiglottis 22.
Epilepsy 226.
Equatorial current 39.
Erysipelas 205.
— migratory 205.
Examination (of body for various occupations) 162.
Excreta 238.
Exercise, bodily 128.
Expectoration 236.
Explosions 166.
Eye disease of newborn children. Trachoma 151. 152. 207.
— Epidemic disease of 206. 207.
— Disease of cornea 206.
— — — conjunctiva 207.
— ball 28.
Eyes 7. 28.
— Cavities of 7. 8. 28.
— Anterior chamber of 31.
— Eye lids 31.
— Muscles of 30.
— Lashes 31.
— Protective arrangements 30. 31.

Face
— ache 171.
— bones of 7. 8.
— cavities of 7. 8.
— sense of sight 28.
Fainting (swooning)
— treating 226.
— revival in case of 226.
Fat 56.
— Law about 140.
Fats 21. 56.
Feather-bed 108.
Feeding grounds, artificially prepared 176.
Fever 23. 184.
— cold 202.
— gastric 193.
— hectic 210.
— puerperal 205.

Fever purulent 205.
— putrid 205.
— spotted 185.
— yellow 203.
Figs 73.
Filter 48. 51.
Fins 209.
Finger 11.
— whitlow 204.
Fish 82. 90. 91.
— Poisoning by 90.
— Preserving of 90.
— roe-cheese 91.
Fissiparous fungi 176.
Flat foot 11.
Flesh (meat) 55. 82.
— bisquit 89.
— broth 86.
— extract 89.
— wild 218.
— inspection of 84. 85.
— kind of 82.
— injurious to health 83—85.
— parasites in 83.
— peptonized 90.
— preparation of 85. 86.
— preserving of 87. 101.
— soup 85.
— white 82.
Flooring 112.
— for bathrooms 112.
— for kitchens 112.
Flour 64.
Fog 39.
Food
— Composition of 54. 55.
— taking 60.
— necessity of 54.
— storage of 101.
— selection of 61.
— coloured diagramm 61.
— Law 139.
— Price calculation for 62.
— Degree of heat of 60.
— children's 150.

Food for a grown-up person 57. 58.
— stuffs 57. 58.
— vessels 100.
Foot wrappings round 107.
— Inflammation of 108.
— Joint 12.
— Perspiration 108.
Forehead 6.
Formaldehyde 182.
Fortress 136.
Fountains
— Wells 46.
— Artesian 46.
— Surface 45.
— Pumping 46.
— Bucket 46.
— Hollow 46.
— Deep 46.
Frost-bites 172.
Fruit 56. 73.
— basket, green 101.
— dried 73.
— jelly 73.
— jam 73.
— sugar 74.
— substitute for 73. 74.
— percentage of water 73.
— wines 94.
Fungi 71.
— edible or poisonous 71. 73.
Fur (pelt) 103.
Furuncle (boil) 204.

Gall
— bile 21. 22.
Game 82.
Ganglion-cells 27.
Gangrene 206.
— by being frozen 172.
— Senile 206.
Gas
— light 123.
— noxious 166.
— poisonous 166.
— saving from suffocation 227. 231.

German measles 185.186.
German silver
— utensils 100.
Girls
— education of 160.
Glanders 208.
Glands 5.
Gluten 56. 63.
Goods
— forbidding import of 147.
— danger through-traffic 148.
Gout 215.
Graham's bread 66.
Grape-sugar 56. 75.
Groin
— bend of the 7.
Growing in of nails 107. 108.
Gymnastic training 159.

Hæmorrhage
— violent of the lungs 210.
Hair on the head 6. 7.
— care of 53.
— capillary vessels 16.
Hand 11.
Hartenstein leguminose 69.
Head 6. 7.
— Erysipelas 205.
— covering of 108.
Health 1.
— Hygiene 1. 2.
— injuries by climate 170.
— injuries through over-exertion of the body 164.
— injuries to by bad stoves 116.
— injuries through weather 146.
— public sanitation 130.
— science of 1. 2.
Hearing 32.
— Auditory bones 32.
— Eustachian canal 32.

Index.

Hearing nerve 32.
— sense of 32.
Heart
— auricles 17.
— beat 237.
— contraction of 18.
— pericardium 15.
— valves, diseases of 18.
— ventricles 18.
— cardiac region 10.
Heat
— apoplexy 173. 174.
— of body 23.
— influence of 170.
— injurious effect of some occupations 164. 165.
— of the air 37. 38.
— stroke 173. 174.
— dry 242.
Heated bags with sand etc. 241. 242.
Heating pans 234.
— apparatus 115. 116.
High fermentation 95.
Hips 7. 11.
Honey
— adulteration of 75.
— cakes 75.
Hops 95.
House
— building of 112. 113.
— colour of 121.
— subsoil and position 109. 110.
— house and kitchen refuse 125. 137.
— filter 49. 50.
— dry-rot 111.
— refuse dry 133.
— — disposal of 133.
— — by burning 133.
Hunger 54.
Hydrophobia 207.
Hygiene
— science of 1.
Hygrometer 37.

Jam 73.
Jaws
— upper 7.

Jaws lower 7.
Ice
— bags 241
— bandages 174.
— bladder 237.
— refrigerator (safes) 102.
Jellies 90.
Immunity 179.
Imperial law
— slaughtering of animals 85.
— for combating infectious diseases 141.
— Vaccination Law 189.
Incandescent light 124.
Incubation
— stage of 184.
India belts 107.
— goods 105.
— rubber 105.
Infant's 149—153.
— food 78.
— cause of crying of 152.
— mortality 149.
Infectious disease 175.
Premilinary conditions of 178.
— authorities 180.
— Course of disease 183.
— Duty of 180.
— Preventive measures 179.
— substances 165.
— Regulations about informing authorities 180.
Infirmaries 142.
Inflammation 204.
Influenza 200.
Ingrowing of the toe-nails 107, 108.
Injections 238.
Injuries by means of occupation 167. 168.
Inoculation against rabies 108.
Insects protection of food against 102.

Inspiration 14.
Insurance
— Invalid 171—173.
Intellectual stimulation 128.
Intermittent fever 202.
Intestine, large 20.
— small 20.
— catarrh 194.
— thorax 12.
— typhoid fever 180.
—al canal 19. 20.
—s of the abdomen 4. 12. 19.
Intoxication 225.
Joints 4.
— diseases of 210.
— grease 5.
— pan 11.
— rheumatism 171.
Iris 29.
Irrigated fields 134.
Irrigotor 218, 238, 239.

Kernel fruit 73.
Kidneys 24.
— inflammation of 187.
Killed by caving in of earth 231.
Kindergarten 153.
Knacker 144.
Knee
— cap 12.
— ham 12.
— joint 12.

Labyrinth 32.
Lachrymal glands 31.
— fluid 31.
Lacrymal dust 8.
Lamps 122.
— shades 124.
Lard 56. 80. 89.
— Law about 140.
Larynx 14.
Lead
— Material containing 139.
— Poisonings through 100. 166.
— Cause of them 100.

Leather for washing 103.
Leaven 64.
Leek 70.
Lemon-juice 92.
— citric acid 92.
Lentils 68.
Leprosy
— Disease of 209.
— Acute 185.
Lettuce salad 70.
Leucamia 214.
Ligaments 4. 5.
Light
— Electric 123. 124.
— beer 95.
— Influence of on germs 122.
— shades 124.
Lighting
— Natural 122.
— Artificial 122.
Lightning stroke 173.
Limbs
— upper 7.
— lower 7. 11. 12.
Linen 103. 104.
Linoleum 113.
Linseed oil 69.
Liqueurs 96.
Liver 21.
— Cod — oil 91.
Loins 7.
Long—sighted 30.
Loss — economic through diseases 1.
Lot system 136.
Low fermentation 95.
Lower jaws 7.
Lunatic asylums 97. 142.
Lungs 12.
— vesicles of 12.
— Pulmonary artery 17.
— — vein 17.
— — consumption 179. 210.
— Pleura pulmonalis 14.
— Great circulation 17.
— Inflammation of 200.
Lupus 211.

Lymph
— Animal 19.
— glands 19.
— Humanized 189.
— Inflammation of 205.
— vessels 19.

Maize 67. 68.
Malaria 172. 202.
Malt (kiln) 95.
— green 95.
Malton wine 95.
Mantle stove 118.
Massage 240.
Mato 98.
Margarine 79. 80. 140.
— cheese 80.
Marrow 4.
Material
— filling up 113.
— porous for cothings 102.
Matter
— boil 204. 205.
— fever (Suppuration) 205.
Mead 75.
Meals 59.
Measles 185.
Measures, State precautionary — for unhealthy occupations 161. 162.
Meat 55. 82.
— Preserved 87.
— Tinned 87.
Medicinal wine 94.
Medicines
— Administering of 239. 240.
Melons 73.
Melted butter 79.
Mercury, poisoning by 166.
Mesentery 19—21.
Met 94.
Metal poisoning 166.
Micro-organisms
— animal 178.
— in water 43. 48.

Middle foot 12.
Milk 56. 76. 77.
— adulterations of 79.
— of diseased animals 77. 212.
— bitter 77.
— blood coloured 77.
— condensed 78.
— cow — as substitute for mother's milk 77. 150.
— curdled 78.
— watery 77.
— freezing of 78.
— for infants 150.
— keeping of 78.
— butter 79.
— Lean (skin) 77.
— preserved 78.
— sugar 56. 74. 76.
— sour 78.
— tooth 60.
— unmatured (biestings) 77.
Millet 68.
Mind, Intellect; 149.
— diseases of brain 213.
— onesided development of 113.
Mineral water 51.
Morphia
— poisoning 225.
Mortality
— in different trades 169.
Mouldy fungi (spores) 178.
Mountain-sickness 40.
Mouth 7.
— cavity of 7—9.
— care of 60.
— water to clean 60.
Movement, voluntary 25.
Mucous membrane 6.
Munich
— mortality in 2.
— decrease of typhoid 180.
Muscarine 72.
Muscles 4.
— muscular rheumatism 171.

Index. 251

Music 128. 159.
Mussels 91.
Mustard plaster 240. 241.
— paper 240.

Nails 6.
— In growing of 107. 108.
Nape 7.
Nature
— enjoying 128.
Necessaries of life 35.
Neck 7.
— Clothing for 105.
Nerves 4. 25—28.
— activity and action 25.
— diseases of 213. 214.
— nervous disorders 171.
— — fever 192.
New-Structures
— beningn 215.
— malignant 215.
Nickel vessels 101.
Nicotine 99.
Nose
— bleeding from 221.
— pharynx 9.
— nasal bone 7.
— — cavity 7. 8.
Nitrogen 35.
Nuisances from factories 137.
Nutritive substances 21. 55.

Oats
— groats 67.
— gruel 67.
Occiput 6.
Occupation, choice of
— unhealthy —s 161.
— Advantages and Disadvantages of special 161.
— women's 161. 162.
Oil 56.
— of mirbane 75.
— fruit 69.
— Poppy oil 69.
— lamps 122.
Oleo-Margarine 80.

Olive oil 69.
— adulterated 69.
Omentum 21.
Onions 70. 92.
Opium
— poisoning by 225.
Optic nerve 28.
Organs of sense 28.
Os sacrum (back of bony pelvis) 10.
Outer garments
— material for 105.
Outfall pipe 126.
Overburdening of school children 157. 158.
Oxalic acid poisoning 224. 225.
Oxidation 36.
Oxygen in the atmosphere 35. 36.
— in the blood 18. 19.
Oysters 91.
Ozone 36.

Painting 240.
Palate 9.
Panaritium (whitlow) 204. 205.
Pancreatic juice 22.
Paraguay tea 98.
Parsley 70.
Pasteur 78. 208.
—ized milk 78.
Pastry 64.
Patent leather 103.
— Earth nut-oil 80.
Peas 68. 70.
— sausage 69.
Peat 126.
Pelvic cavity 11.
Pelvis 7. 10.
Periosteum 4.
Perspiration 23.
— development 243.
Petroleum 123.
— lamps 122.
— Imperial Law concerning 139.
Phosphorus (poisoning by) 166. 225.
Pickled (smoked) beef 88.

Pine apple 73.
Pipe well 46.
Plague 202. 303.
— bubonic 202. 203.
— lung 202. 203.
— Asiatic 202. 203.
Plasma 15.
Poisoning 224—226.
— by means of verdigris 100.
— metals 166.
— phosphorus 166.
— fungi 71—73.
Poisons 177. 224. 225.
Polar-current 39.
Polenta 68.
Polluting of rivers 133.
Pollution (contamination) 135.
Pomatum 53.
Poor
— Provision for the poor and sick 141.
Posterior orifice 20.
Potatoes 56. 69.
— brandy 96.
— Preservation of 101.
Poultices 54.
Predisposition 178. 179.
Premonitory symptons (Prodromal stage) of disease 184.
Preparation of food 58. 59.
Pressure
— sensation of 33.
Priessnitz swathings 242.
Propagation 34.
— of infections 148.
Prosperity 138.
Protecting apparatus 222. 223.
Pulsation, number of 18.
— in invalids 237.
Pulse (leguminose) 68.
Pulses 55. 68.
Pump-well 46.
Pumpernickel (black bread) 65. 66.
Pupil (of the eye) 28.
Purification
— Self — of rivers 48.

Pyrolus 19. 20.
Pyronylic acid 92.

Quarantine by sea 147.
Quinces 73.

Rabies 221.
Rachitis 153.
Radishes 70. 73. 92.
Radius 11.
Railways 145.
— Regulations concerning 146.
Raisins 73.
— wine 94.
Rapeseed-oil 123.
Recreation 128.
— places for 137.
Rectum 20.
Red wine 93. 94.
Refreshment 59.
— luxury 93. 95.
Refuse as manure 133. 134.
— Removal of 125, 131.
— Final destruction 133.
Regulations in factories about working 163.
— workrooms 163
Remittent fever 191.
— typhus 192. 194.
Removal of foreign objects, insects etc. 231.
— of refuse 131.
— of waste water from factories 134.
Respiration, artificial 230.
Retina 29.
Retrograde movement of people 149.
Revival
— efforts in case of frozen people 172.
— in other accidents 224.
Rheumatism 171.
Rhum 96.
Ribs 10.
— Pleura costalis 14.
Rice 67.
Rickets 153.

Ringworm 208.
Roasting of food 58. 59.
Roentgen rays 222.
Roofs of tiles 121.
— from cardboard strongly tarred 112.
— wood-cement 112.
— wood 121.
— materials for 112.
— Rooms under 127.
— Regulations concerning use of rooms under 127.
— straw 121.
— Metal 121.
Ruptures 106. 223.
Rye 66. 68.
— brandy 96.
— bread 66.

Saccharine law 74.
Sale of food 138.
Saliva
— glands 9.
Salts 56.
Sand filter 50. 51.
Sauerkraut 71.
Sausages 88. 89.
— colouring of 89.
— poisoning by 89. 194.
Scab 208.
Scarlet fever 185—187.
Schlempe 96.
Scholars, pupil suicide 159.
School
— lesson 157.
— physicians 153. 159.
— benches 156.
— education 149.
— house 154. 155.
— time 153. 154.
— room 154—156.
— compulsory 149.
Sciatica 171.
Scrofulosis 211.
Sea ports
— water 51.
— Watching of health in 147.
Seasonings 59. 91. 92.

Seasons
— relations to certain diseases 174. 175.
Secret (keeping — of remedies)
— Patent medicines 141.
— diseases on ships 147.
Sellery 70.
Sensations of pain 35.
— of touch 33.
— sensory nerves 25. 33.
Sense of pressure contact 33.
— perception of 35.
Serum 15. 179.
Sesame oil 69. 79.
Settlement 131.
— community 130.
Sewage (tuns, buckets) 127.
Sewers with pipes 132.
Shell-fish 91.
— fruit 73.
Shin-bone 12.
Ships
— sanitary condition of 145.
— bisquit 66.
Shoes 107.
Shoulder
— blade 11.
— joint 11.
Shortsightedness 30. 155.
Sick
— bed 233. 234.
— care of 239.
— conduct with 236.
— Hospital 142 192. 233.
— insurance 167. 168.
— isolation of 141. 180.
— room 233.
— support 167. 168.
— transport of 243.
Silicious marl 50.
Silk stuffs 103.
Sinews 5.
Siphon 126. 139.
Sitting bone 11.
Skeleton 4.
Skin 4. 6.
— care of the 53.

Skin diseases of 208. 209. 211.
— grease 6.
— noxious remedies for 53.
— sclerotic of eye 28.
— upper (epidermis) 6.
Skull 6.
— cavity (cranial) of 7.
— bone 7.
Sleep 33.
— want of 33.
— duration of 33.
Small-pox 185. 187. 188. 193—199.
Smell
— olfactory nerves 33.
— sense of 33.
Smoked meat 88.
Snails 91
Snake-bites 221.
Snuff 99.
Soap 51.
Social intercourse 129.
Society 130.
Soft constituents of body 4.
Soldier's rye bread 66.
Sound-vibrations 32.
Soup for infants 150.
— tablets 89.
Sour milk 78.
Soxhlet's apparatus 78.
Spanish fly-paper 241.
Spectacles 30.
Speech 14. 15.
— development of 152. 153.
Spelt 66.
Spices 59.
Spinage 70.
Spinal column 10.
Spirilli (bacilli) 176.
Spitoon 212. 213.
— in school—room 155.
Spleen 19. 24.
Spores (bacilli) 176.
Sprains 223.
Spring water 44. 45.
— aqueducts 45.
— pollution of 45.
— s mineral 45.

Squinting 30.
Standing 152. 164.
Starch 21. 56.
— syrup 74.
— sugar 74.
— molasses 74.
Statistics of diseases and deaths in different occupations 169.
Steam heating—apparatus 121.
Stearine 80.
Steep writing 157.
Sterilized milk 78.
Sticking plaster 218.
Stiff neck
— epidemic 201.
Stockings
— garters 107.
Stomach 19. 20.
— pump, application of 225.
— catarrh 193, 194.
— gastric juice 22.
— pit of 10.
Stone fruit 73.
Storage rooms for food etc. 101.
Stove 116—121.
— heating 116—118.
— dampers 118.
— Iron 116.
Stoves
— Filled 118.
Street cleaning 135.
— sprinkling 135.
Stretcher 243.
Strychnine
— poisoning by 225.
Stupefaction 225.
Stye 206.
Subterranean air 44.
— water 44.
— — precautions against in houses 110.
Suffocation
— saving from 229.
Suicide of school boys 159.
Sugar 56. 74. 92.
— candy 74.
— containing 21.

Sugar ware for children 151.
Sunday rest 163.
Sunlight 122.
Sunstroke 173. 174.
Surface water 47.
— artificial purification of 48—51.
Swallowing of foreign bodies 231.
Swathings cold 241. 242.
Sweat 6. 24.
— ing cures 242.
Sweet stuffs 74. 75.
— wines 93.
— Laws about them 74. 140.
Swiss tapeworm 90.
Swollen veins 108.
— varicose veins 108.
Syphilis 209.
System of pails 127.

Table oils 92.
— oesophagus 19. 20. 22.
Tallow 89.
Tapeworm 84. 85.
— of dog 209. 216.
— Echinococcus 209. 216.
Tar—soap 53.
Tart 66.
Taste
— Sense of 33.
Tea 97—99.
Teacher
— duties towards children 153.
Teeth 4. 9.
— cutting of 152.
— maladies (bakers and and confectioners) 165.
— crown of 9.
— care of 60. 61.
— powder 60.
— ache 242.
— root of 9.
Temperature 33.
Temples 6.

Tendon of Achilles 12.
Theatre 141. 159.
Thermometer 38.
— clinical 237.
— maximal 237.
Thigh 11.
— bone 11.
— joint 12.
Thumb 11.
Thunderstorm
— influence of 36.
Thymol soap 53.
Tight lacing (Corsets, stays) 106. 107.
Tissue
— adipose 4.
Toa-foo 69.
Tobacco 99. 100.
— smoking in schools 158.
Toes 11. 12.
Tongue 9. 22.
Tonsilitis 197—199.
Tonsils 9.
— swelling of the 186.
Tourniquet 221.
Trachoma 207.
Trade
— inspector 161.
— Law concerning industrial occupations 162. 163. 167.
Traffic 144—147.
Train oil 91.
Transport of injured persons 222. 243.
Travelling 145. 146.
Trichina 83. 85. 209.
— microscopic investigation of pork for trichina 85.
Tropical fever 202.
Trunk 10.
— Chest 12.
— Chest-bone 10.
— Pleurisy 14. 200. 201.
— Cavity of the chest (Thorax) 10.
— cavities 10.
Trusses 107.
Tuberculosis

Tuberculosis bacilli 209.
— General (Miliar) 211.
— memorandum on 212.
— crowned with the price-pamphlet 212.
— various forms of 210.
— curable nature of 211.
— dissemination of and protectiv measures against 212.
Tumours
— encysted 215.
— benign 215.
— turf-springs 45.
Turnips, Beetroot 70.
Tympanic cavity 32.
Tympanum 32.
Typhoid 179. 190.
— Hunger 190.
— War or famine 190.
Typhus 190.

Ulcers 107.
— on the conjunctiva 206.
— on skin 209.
— in the stomach 337.
Ulna 11. 27.
Undergarments 104.105.
Understanding (reason)
— awakening of 153.
Unions 130.
Upper arm bone 11.
— — head 11.
Upper jaws 7.
Urine
— canal 24.
— excretion of 24.
— glass 238.
— organs 19.
Uvula 9.

Vaccination 188—190.
— against smallpox 188—190.
— injured through 190.
Varioloids 188.

Vegetable poison 225.
Vegetables 69—71.
— dried 71.
— fresh 69—71.
— percentage of water in 70.
— tablets 71.
— veins 15. 16.
— wheels 115.
Vermiform
— contimation (intestine) of 20.
Venæ cavæ 16.
Ventilation 114. 115.
— artificial 115.
— natural 110. 115.
— stove 119.
— arrangements 122.
— pipes 127.
Verdigris
— poisoning by 100.
Vessels for food 100.
— iron 101.
— enamelled 101.
Vestibule (of the ear) 32.
Vibrions 176.
Vinegar 92.
Virulence of germs
— of disease 178.
Viscera (Entrails) 4. 12.
— of the abdomen 19.
— thorax, trunk 12.
Visual power
— injury through various occupations 164.
— Pupil of the eye 29.
Vitreous humour (of the eye) 28.
Vocal cords 15.
Voice 14.
Vomiting 239.

Walking 152. 154.
Wall, building material of 110.
— paper in dwelling-rooms 113.
— poisonous 114. 128.
— heavy materials 114.
Walls as protection
— against heat 121.

Water 35. 42. 56.
— hard and soft 43.
— meteoric 44.
— boiling of 49.
— chicken pox 190.
— filter 49.
— beds 235.
— cures 53. 54.
— rabies 207.
— bandages 222. 237. 241.
— use of 135.
— supply by aquæducts 135. 136.
Watercress 70.
Weather change of 39.
— influence on 164. 165. 170.
Well
— Bucket 46.
— Pump 46.
Wells
— deep water 46.

Wheat 66. 67.
Wheaten bread 66. 67.
Whey
— cures 80. 81.
Whiskey 96.
White wine 94.
Whitewash 181.
Whitlow 204.
Whooping cough 199.
Wild cherry
— poisoning by 225.
Wind
— wheels 39. 40. 115.
— strength of 39.
Windows
— size in proportion to size of rooms 122.
— curtains 121. 122.
Wine 93. 94.
— Law 140.
Woolen clothing 102— to 105.

Work, children's 161. 162.
Worm 204.
Wounds
— treatment of 217. 218.
— antiseptic 204.
— gangrene 205.
— disease of 203. 204.
— germs of 204.
— tetanus 206.
— through cutting 217.
Writer's cramp 164.
Yeast
— fungi 64.
— bacteria 177.

Zine-vessels 101. 139. 140.
— containing 139. 140.
— Law obout use of 139. 140.

MIX
Papier aus verantwortungsvollen Quellen
Paper from responsible sources
FSC® C105338

If you have any concerns about our products,
you can contact us on
ProductSafety@springernature.com

In case Publisher is established outside the EU,
the EU authorized representative is:
**Springer Nature Customer Service Center GmbH
Europaplatz 3, 69115 Heidelberg, Germany**

Printed by Libri Plureos GmbH
in Hamburg, Germany